T0296865

An Introduction to Male Reproductive Medicine

An Introduction to Male Reproductive Medicine

Edited by

Craig Niederberger, MD, FACS

Clarence C. Saelhof Professor and Head, Department of Urology,
University of Illinois, Chicago, College of Medicine, and Professor,
Department of Bioengineering, University of Illinois, Chicago,
College of Engineering, Chicago, IL, USA

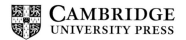

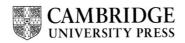

Shaftesbury Road, Cambridge CB2 8EA, United Kingdom

One Liberty Plaza, 20th Floor, New York, NY 10006, USA

477 Williamstown Road, Port Melbourne, VIC 3207, Australia

314–321, 3rd Floor, Plot 3, Splendor Forum, Jasola District Centre, New Delhi – 110025, India

103 Penang Road, #05–06/07, Visioncrest Commercial, Singapore 238467

Cambridge University Press is part of Cambridge University Press & Assessment,
a department of the University of Cambridge.

We share the University's mission to contribute to society through the pursuit of
education, learning and research at the highest international levels of excellence.

www.cambridge.org
Information on this title: www.cambridge.org/9780521173025

First published 2011

A catalogue record for this publication is available from the British Library

Library of Congress Cataloging-in-Publication data
An introduction to male reproductive medicine / edited by Craig Niederberger.
    p. ; cm.
  Includes bibliographical references and index.
  ISBN 978-0-521-17302-5 (Paperback)
1. Infertility, Male.   I. Niederberger, Craig S., 1960– editor.
  [DNLM: 1. Infertility, Male. WJ 709]
  RC889.I62 2011
  616.6′92–dc22   2010045952

ISBN   978-0-521-17302-5   Paperback

Contents

The color plate section can be found between pages 120 and 121.

Contributors

Robert E. Brannigan, MD
Associate Professor, Department of Urology, Northwestern University,
Feinberg School of Medicine, Chicago, IL, USA

Ettore Caroppo, MD
Reproductive Unit and Andrology Outpatients Clinic,
ASL BARI, PO "F. Iaia", Conversano (Ba), Italy

Grace M. Centola, PhD, HCLD (ABB)
President, Cryobank Compliance Services, Rochester, NY, USA

Randall B. Meacham, MD
Professor and Chief, Division of Urology, The University of Colorado
School of Medicine, Denver, CO, USA

Craig Niederberger, MD, FACS
Clarence C. Saelhof Professor and Head,
Department of Urology, University of Illinois, Chicago,
College of Medicine, and
Professor, Department of Bioengineering,
University of Illinois, Chicago, College of Engineering,
Chicago, IL, USA

Bradley J. Van Voorhis, MD
Professor of Reproductive Endocrinology, and Director,
Division of Reproductive Endocrinology and Infertility,
University of Iowa Carver College of Medicine, Iowa City, IA, USA

Moshe Wald, MD
Assistant Professor, Department of Urology, University of Iowa,
Iowa City, IA, USA

Daniel H. Williams IV, MD
Assistant Professor, Department of Urology,
University of Wisconsin School of Medicine and Public Health,
Madison, WI, USA

Preface

Few medical fields are moving as fast as male infertility. Current treatment for a patient experiencing difficulty impregnating his partner bears only a fair resemblance to therapies of even two decades ago. This rapid progress is in part influenced by parallel advances in female reproductive medicine, such as the development of technology that allows a single sperm injected into an ovum to yield a baby. Nevertheless, even by itself, male reproductive medicine over the past few years has been a rushing current of innovations in medical treatment and surgery.

Evaluation and treatment of the infertile male can appear to be an arcane, confusing maze. Male reproductive problems are not rare events that only an occasional physician will encounter; a male factor causes infertility in couples as often as a female factor does. We wrote this book to help you unravel the mysteries of male infertility and to prepare you to treat the patient who has difficulty impregnating his partner. The fourth edition of *Infertility in the Male* is an excellent reference text, but at nearly 700 dense pages, it can be challenging to navigate when you're first beginning to see and treat male patients. This book is a companion to that reference text, including pointers to locations with expanded discussions of salient topics.

Each chapter in this book is written by a single author who will take you through one of the eight basic components of male reproductive medicine: biology, clinical evaluation, surgery, medicine, immunology, genetics, semen analysis, and integration with care for the female. All are designed to be easy to read. We don't shy away from our opinions; when you see patients you ultimately have to make decisions, and opinions form the basis for those choices. We are describing how we evaluate and treat infertile men, providing our reasoning, and pointing you to fuller explanations in the fourth edition of *Infertility in the Male*. As you progress in learning this field, we hope you will read the reference text, as you may come to your own, reasoned opinions about the best way to approach an infertile man.

The fundamental intent of this book is to be an accessible entry into the field of male reproductive medicine. Enjoy the book, and welcome to one of the most interesting and gratifying areas of medicine.

Male reproductive medicine: anatomy and physiology

Ettore Caroppo, MD

Introduction

Reproduction is a highly specialized function of a healthy living organism. This concept may sound ordinary and simplistic, but it needs to be emphasized at a time when reproduction is undervalued by many who consider it a matter pertaining exclusively to sperm and eggs. As a result, it is a great achievement that the World Health Organization (WHO), when releasing its *Glossary of Terminology in Assisted Reproduction*, has defined infertility as **a disease of the reproductive system** [1], raising it to a level that clinicians have the responsibility to treat.

Treating male infertility means treating people not cells. Although assisted reproduction techniques may represent a solution for some infertile couples with male factor infertility, when a doctor is faced with an infertile male patient, he or she has the duty to try to improve and if possible restore their reproductive health.

Understanding the physiology of the male reproductive system results in a better understanding of the physiopathology of male infertility. This is also the basis of learning how to manage an infertile male patient.

Anatomy

It may be surprising, but the male reproductive system does not only comprise the testes, the accessory glands, and the penis, but also the brain and other structures located in the cranium (Figure 1.1). Before involving the genitourinary tract, reproduction depends on the interplay between neural and endocrine

An Introduction to Male Reproductive Medicine, ed. Craig Niederberger. Published by Cambridge University Press. © Cambridge University Press 2011.

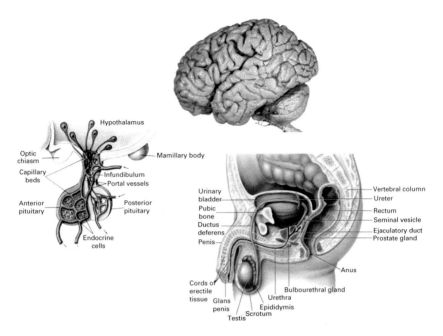

Figure 1.1 Anatomy of the male reproductive system.

events. The **brain** determines the timing of onset of puberty but also controls parenting behavior: a child may be first conceived in his/her parent's brain. A crucial role in controlling sexual behavior and reproduction is played by the **hypothalamus**, the ventral-most part of the diencephalon, which is located on either side of the third ventricle, with the hypothalamic sulcus delineating its dorsal border. It extends from the rostral limit of the optic chiasm to the caudal limit of the mamillary bodies.

The first impulse to spermatogenesis and secretion of sex hormones arises from the arcuate nucleus, located in the tuberal region of the hypothalamus, which contains many of the neurons that control the endocrine functions of the adenohypophysis. Terminals of gonadotropin-releasing hormone (GnRH)-secreting neurons release their secretions in the median eminence and infundibulum, where they enter the **hypophyseal portal system**. This is a capillary network originating from the superior hypophyseal arteries, which recombines in long portal veins draining down the pituitary stalk to the anterior lobe, when it breaks up into another capillary network and re-forms into venous channels. GnRH is then driven to the anterior pituitary, a gland originating from Rathke's pouch that lies in the sella turcica, precisely to the gonadotrophs, basophil-staining cells, which constitute 10%–15% of anterior pituitary cells and are located throughout the entire anterior lobe The gonadotrophs synthesize follicle-stimulating hormone (FSH) and luteinizing hormone (LH) and release them into the systemic circulation; both hormones reach the **testis** by testicular arteries. The arterial supply to the testes follows the lobular division of seminiferous tubules, so that each lobulus is supplied by one recurrent artery; segmental arteries and capillaries become branched between the Leydig cells and then give rise to the venous system. The pattern of blood supply to the testis is also essential for maintaining a lower testicular temperature compared with body temperature. In the pampiniform plexus, the convoluted testicular artery is surrounded by several veins coiling around the artery many times, so arterial blood is cooled down by surrounding venous blood.

The testis measures 15–25 cm^3 in volume. It is surrounded by a fibrous capsule, the tunica albuginea, from which septations extend toward the testicular mediastinum, dividing the testis into 200–300 lobules. Each of these lobules contains several highly convoluted seminiferous tubules. Each seminiferous tubule consists of a basement membrane lined by Sertoli cells, interspersed with germ cells at various stages of maturation. Seminiferous tubules arise and end at the rete testis, which is an anastomosing network of tubules that empties into the **efferent ductules**. Spermatozoa are then transported through efferent ductules into a single duct, the **epididymis**, and then enter the **vas deferens**, which propels its contents by peristaltic motion into the ejaculatory ducts. These receive fluid from the **seminal vesicles** (two large lobulated glands 5–10 cm in length), which lie inferiorly and dorsally to the bladder wall. They consist of blind-coiled alveoli with several diverticuli; their secretions make up 1.5–2 ml of the average 3 ml ejaculate and provide fructose, prostaglandins, and coagulating proteins. The ejaculatory ducts terminate in the prostatic urethra, where 30–50 tubuloalveolar glands forming the **prostate** open. The prostate is inferior to the bladder and surrounds the proximal portion of the urethra, where it emerges from the bladder. The prostate averages 3.4 cm in length, 4.4 cm in width, and 2.6 cm in depth. It is divided by the urethra and ejaculatory ducts into three major zones: peripheral zone (comprising about 70% of the glandular prostate); central zone (accounting for approximately 20% of the glandular prostate); and transition zone (represents 5% of the prostatic tissue). The prostatic contribution to the ejaculate is approximately 0.5 ml, and it is rich in citrate, zinc, polyamines, cholesterol, prostaglandins, and various proteases important in the liquefaction of semen. Fluid is also added to the seminal plasma by the **bulbourethral glands** and **glands of Littré** during its transit through the penile urethra.

The **penis** is built by paired crura forming the corpora cavernosa and by the bulb containing the urethra and becoming the corpus spongiosum, which is expanded at the tip to the glans. At the base of the penis the corpora cavernosa are covered by the ischiocavernosus muscles, whose contractions, under the control of the pudendal nerve, enhance penile rigidity, and the corpus spongiosum is surrounded by the bulbocavernosus muscle, whose contractions are involved in the ejaculation. Blood supply to the penis is provided by a dorsal superficial and cavernosal arterial system, derived from the internal pudendal artery, which gives off a perineal branch and continues as the penile artery; additional blood supply may be found in the form of accessory pudendal arteries. The deep penile arteries enter the crura cavernosa and stream on both sides centrally within the corpora cavernosa. The coiled helicine arteries then directly supply the sinusoidal spaces, and the smaller arteries travel between the trabeculae. Subtunical venous plexus collect blood from the sinusoidal spaces, leading into emissary veins, which drain into spongiosal veins, circumflex veins, or directly into the deep dorsal vein and further into cavernosal and crural veins ending in the internal pudendal vein. The retrocoronal plexus drains the glans penis into the deep dorsal vein, which finally enters the periprostatic venous plexus.

Embryology

This section will briefly review the embryology of the male reproductive system, whose knowledge is required to understand the physiopathology of cryptorchidism and of hypospadias. A more detailed description of this argument can be found in [2] (chapters 1 and 6).

Testis development begins during the fifth week of gestation, but remains undifferentiated for the first 2 weeks. It arises from a mix of mesothelium, mesenchyme, and primordial germ cells, and becomes apparent with the formation of the gonadal ridge, which is composed by the epithelial layer (cortex) and the mesenchymal area (medulla). **By the sixth week Sertoli cells develop from the medullar sex cord under the influence of the sex-determining region of the Y chromosome (SRY), and start producing anti-Müllerian hormone (AMH), which will halt the development of the paramesonephric ducts.** Between the eighth and 10th week of development, seminiferous cords are separated by mesenchyme, which is stimulated to become Leydig cells by SRY proteins. Leydig cells start producing testosterone, initially under the stimulation of placental chorionic gonadotropins, but eventually the embryo's own hypothalamic–pituitary axis takes over control with the pituitary secretion of human chorionic gonadotropin (hCG). **Testosterone's effect is the development of the mesonephric duct in the Wolffian duct.** The distal portion of the Wolffian duct becomes the vas deferens. Near the urogenital sinus, a pair of lateral buds develops from the duct and become the seminal vesicles. The most cranial of the duct will disintegrate and remnant tissue will form the appendix epididymis, while the mesonephric tubules that grew near developing testes will become incorporated into the testis–epididymis structure as efferent ductules.

The **descent of the testis is a complex, multistage process requiring interaction of anatomical and hormonal factors**. The testis descends from an intraabdominal location into the bottom of the scrotum in two major phases, the transabdominal and the inguinoscrotal descent [3]. This two-stage process is guided by two mesenteric ligaments: the cranial suspensory ligament and the caudal genitoinguinal ligament or gubernaculums. The first stage occurs between 10 and 23 weeks of gestation. Initially, the undifferentiated gonads are attached to the abdominal wall in a pararenal position. Cranial suspensory ligament attaches the gonad to the posterior abdominal wall, whereas gubernaculums connects the testis via the epididymis to the future intraabdominal inner ring of the inguinal canal. Under the effects of hormones, cranial suspensory ligament regresses, whereas gubernaculums develops its caudal segment into the gubernacular bulb, a reaction called the "swelling reaction," protruding into the forming scrotal sac. The swelling reaction of the gubernaculum holds the testis very close to the future internal inguinal ring, which causes the transabdominal migration of the testes into the inguinal region. The second, inguinoscrotal, phase occurs between 26 and 28 weeks of gestation, when the testes move from the inguinal region to the scrotum. This phase is due to shortening of the gubernacular cord and outgrowth of the gubernacular bulb. There is no consensus about the factor regulating the two phases of testicular descent; nevertheless, androgens play an important role in this matter.

External genitalia begin their development in an undifferentiated state: the presence of Y chromosome with *Sry* gene and the synthesis of testosterone will drive differentiation to a male phenotype. The first step is the formation of the genital tubercle from the mesenchyme, which will subsequently elongate and become the phallus. Additional proliferating tissue on either side of the cloacal membrane forms the labioscrotal swelling and the urogenital folds. In the presence of testosterone, the phallus lengthens and enlarges to form the penis. The urethral groove, originating from the urogenital membrane of the cloaca, grows as well: more medial endodermal folds will fuse in the ventral midline to form the urethra; the more lateral ectodermal folds will fuse over the developing urethra to form the penile shaft skin and prepuce. As these two layers fuse from posterior to anterior, they leave behind a skin line, the median raphe. By 13 weeks, the urethra is almost complete. A ring of ectoderm forms just proximal to the developing glans penis. This skin advances over the corona glandis and eventually covers the glans entirely as prepuce or foreskin.

A brief introduction to the regulation of hormone secretion and action

Feedback regulation

The endocrine glands constituting the hypothalamus–pituitary–gonadal axis do not continuously synthesize and secrete their hormones in a shower fashion. On the contrary, one distinctive feature of hormone secretion through the hypothalamus–pituitary–gonadal axis is that they regulate their own secretion through negative feedback inhibition. What this means is that a hormone (testosterone) secreted from a peripheral gland (the testis) binds to its receptor on cells in the hypothalamus and hypophysis, and inhibits the secretion of tropic hormones (GnRH and LH). Less GnRH secretion leads to less LH secretion, which leads to less stimulation of testosterone secretion by Leydig cells. Depending on the distance taken by hormones to deliver their feedback message to its destination, there are three kinds of feedback: long loop feedback, short loop feedback, and ultrashort loop feedback (Figure 1.2).

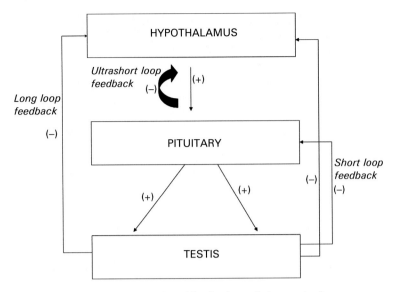

Figure 1.2 Schematic representation of feedback regulation mechanisms.

The usefulness of negative feedback inhibition is that it results in hormonal homeostasis, which is the maintenance of hormone levels within a particular appropriate physiologic range. In the case of a damaged testis, a decreased secretion of testosterone would be expected; however, the homeostatic model would bring testosterone back up towards its normal daily level of secretion, as lower testosterone levels would lead to a consequent decrease in the degree of negative feedback inhibition on the hypothalamus and anterior pituitary. In addition, the release from negative feedback inhibition would lead to an increase in GnRH and LH secretion, and more LH will stimulate the healthy testis to secrete more testosterone.

Downregulation, upregulation, and desensitization

Apart from the feedback pathway of hormone secretion control, other important factors affecting the response to hormone stimuli are downregulation or upregulation of receptor levels and desensitization. **The downregulation mechanism is intended to prevent an excessive response to a higher-than-normal hormone level.** The exposure of testicular cells expressing the endogenous LH receptor (LHR) to a high concentration of hCG or LH downregulates the levels of cell surface receptor. Concomitant with the downregulation of cell surface LHR, a decrease in the abundance of all LHR mRNA transcripts is observed. An important clinical application of this mechanism is that an excessive exogenous hormone administration in order to increase target gland activity will be useless, as it will lead to a downregulation of hormone receptors. **Instead, upregulation occurs when an increase in receptor level is required**: an example of upregulation in the testis is the permissive role of FSH on LH–Leydig cell interaction: FSH stimulates Sertoli cells to secrete insulin-like growth factor (IGF)-1, which acts to induce LHRs, leading to an enhancement in steroidogenesis.

Desensitization is an important component of the regulation of hormone actions and can occur at multiple levels. For example, very old experiments demonstrated the existence of two steps in the steroidogenic pathway that contribute to the desensitization of steroidogenic responses observed in male rats injected with LH/CG, or in freshly isolated rat or mouse Leydig cells or cultured Leydig tumor cells exposed to LH/CG. These include a reduction in the activity and/or levels of 17α-hydroxylase/17,20-lyase and a reduction in the amount of cholesterol available for steroidogenesis [4], so that an excessive LH/hCG-stimulated testosterone secretion is prevented.

Autocrine, paracrine, and endocrine regulation

The sophisticated control of hormone synthesis and release involves also mechanisms played at autocrine, paracrine, and endocrine levels. Autocrine control is applied when a hormone controls its own secretion through local action on the cell in which it is produced. Paracrine control is a form of bioregulation in which secretion produced by one cell type in a tissue diffuses through the tissue and affects another cell type in the same tissue. Endocrine control is modulated by hormones secreted by other glands, transported through the bloodstream to the target gland, where they play their modulating role.

Hypothalamus–pituitary–gonadal axis

The following sections will focus on the hypothalamus–pituitary–gonadal axis hormone pattern and regulation of secretion. Figure 1.3 and Table 1.1 summarize the concepts exposed below. For a more detailed description of this argument, please refer to [2] (chapter 2).

Gonadotropin-releasing hormone

GnRH is a decapeptide produced in the GnRH neurons and released in the portal blood in discrete pulses. It has been demonstrated that the frequency and amplitude of GnRH stimulation provide signals for the differential regulation of LH and FSH secretion. At higher GnRH pulse frequencies, LH secretion increases disproportionately more than FSH secretion, whereas at lower GnRH pulse frequencies, FSH secretion is favored. In particular, LH-β subunit RNA levels seem to be stimulated by a GnRH pulse frequency every 120 minutes. The pattern of GnRH pulsatile secretion seems to be intrinsic to GnRH neurons. GnRH neurons have been found to display rhythmic activity in multiple time domains, ranging from burst firing on the order of seconds to episodes of increased firing rate that occur on the order of many minutes.

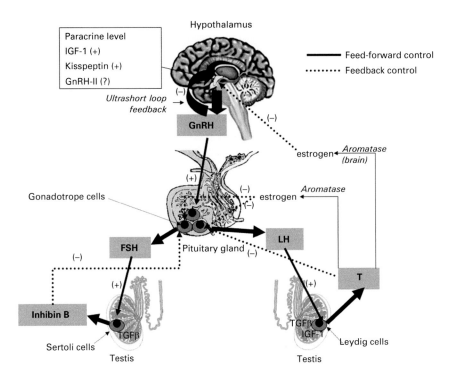

Figure 1.3 Schematic representation of human hypothalamus–pituitary–testis axis. FSH, follicle-stimulating hormone; GnRH, gonadotropin-releasing hormone; IGF, insulin growth factor; LH, luteinizing hormone; T, testosterone; TGF, transforming growth factor.

GnRH is able to regulate its own release (*autocrine regulation*) by means of an ultrashort loop feedback mechanism [5]. GnRH neurons are able to activate and suppress their own activity using GnRH itself as an intra-GnRH neural network signal, a strategy that could have important implications for generation of the GnRH surge in addition to the regulation of pulsatile release. As a matter of fact, a substantial subpopulation of adult GnRH neurons expresses GnRH receptors (GnRHR-1), which can be inhibited by a low dose of GnRH. GnRH neurons could also modulate their own secretion through the synthesis of factors other than GnRH, such as endocannabinoids.

Regulation of GnRH secretion, however, does not only apply to GnRH neurons. A *paracrine control* of GnRH secretion has been postulated, involving the role of a second GnRH subtype, GnRH-II, which differs from GnRH (also called GnRH-I) by three amino acid residues. The actual role of GnRH-II is still to be established: a role in reproductive behavior has been suggested, but it has been also found to stimulate FSH and LH release, probably via the GnRH-I pathway. In addition, IGF-1 may be involved in the paracrine control of GnRH secretion, directly acting on GnRH neurons in the hypothalamus to enhance GnRH gene transcription and play a crucial role in controlling the onset of

Table 1.1 Regulation of hypothalamic–pituitary–gonadal axis hormone release

Hormone	Autocrine regulation	Paracrine regulation	Endocrine regulation
GnRH	GnRH itself (−)	GnRH II (+), IGF-1 (+), kisspeptin (+)	Testosterone (−), estrogens (−), neurotensin (+), norepinephrine (+)
FSH	−	Activin (+), follistatin (−)	GnRH (+), estrogens (−), inhibin B (−)
LH		Activin (+), follistatin (−)	GnRH (+), testosterone (−)
Testosterone	−	IGF-1 (+), GH(+), CRH (−), TGF-β (−), IL-1α (±)	LH (+)

+ Stimulatory effect, − Inhibitory effect. Transforming growth factor-β (TGF-β), corticotropin-releasing hormone (CRH), interleukin 1α (IL-1α), growth hormone (GH), insulin-like growth factor 1 (IGF-1).

puberty. Finally, kisspeptin, the RF-amide peptide ligand, may be involved in the paracrine control of GnRH release.

Testosterone, through its aromatization to estradiol, plays an important role in the *endocrine regulation of GnRH secretion*. Estradiol orchestrates the activity patterns of several neurotransmitter systems within the GnRH network to bring about the GnRH surge; it uses the excitatory amino acids neurotensin and norepinephrine to activate GnRH electrical activity at the level of the GnRH cell body, and neuropeptide Y at the level of GnRH terminals, and reduces the β-endorphin neurons level of activity to disinhibit GnRH neurons. Estradiol is also supposed to influence GnRH pulse generator function: experiments on brain slice preparation demonstrated that it reduces the frequency of GnRH secretion through a pathway involving GABAergic neurons.

Gonadotropins

Gonadotropins FSH and LH are glycoproteins consisting of a common α-subunit and a hormone-specific β-subunit, which are associated through noncovalent interactions. While the β-subunits determine the functional specificity of gonadotropins, **their intrinsic bioactivity is largely determined by their degree of glycosylation. In each blood sample, at least 20–30 different FSH isoforms can be separated by electrophoresis. Weakly glycosylated forms of the hormones have a short circulatory half-time, and although totally deglycosylated gonadotropins are able to interact with their cognate receptor, they are unable to evoke**

generation of a second messenger signal. Highly glycosylated isoforms (acidic) display longer elimination half-life and stronger biologic power.

Gonadotropins are essential for spermatogenesis and secretion of testicular androgens: lack of gonadotropin results in suppression of spermatogenesis, as demonstrated by hypophysectomy, by GnRH immunization, and by GnRH analog treatment. Both FSH and LH play an important role in regulating spermatogenesis. FSH is essential to promote spermatogenesis in men, as it maintains normal testicular size, seminiferous tubular diameter, and sperm number and motility: inactivating FSH mutation or inactivation of FSH receptor gene lead to spermatogenic failure. LH participates in regulating spermatogenesis by stimulating the synthesis of testosterone, which plays an essential role in spermatid maturation: inactivation of LH was found to cause arrest of spermatogenesis and absence of Leydig cells. A permissive role of FSH is postulated, as FSH-stimulated Sertoli cells to secrete IGF-1, which acts in an autocrine and paracrine fashion to induce LHRs and enhance proliferation and steroidogenesis in mice Leydig cells. LH is secreted primarily in pulses: GnRH secretory bursts are followed uniformly by a slightly time-delayed pulse of LH secretion. LH pulses occur in an ultradian fashion, with a mean frequency of approximately one event per hour or one every 90–120 min [6]. On the contrary, FSH secretion is predominantly basal, and it seems to be not directly coupled to GnRH pulses.

Regulation of gonadotropin secretion in the human involves a complex interplay between feed-forward stimulation by GnRH from the hypothalamus, feedback control by sex steroids and inhibin from the testes, and, probably, autocrine/paracrine modulation by other factors within the pituitary. The pattern of GnRH feed-forward regulation of gonadotropin secretion has been illustrated in the previous section. Members of the transforming growth factor (TGF)-β superfamily, activin, inhibin, and follistatin, are produced in the anterior pituitary and seem to be involved in the paracrine/autocrine regulation of FSH secretion. Testosterone feedback control activity at the pituitary level can be direct (mediated by its binding to the androgen receptor [AR]) as well as indirect (mediated by aromatization to estrogens and binding to pituitary estrogen receptors). Testosterone exerts a direct feedback control of LH secretion, while its action on FSH secretion is mostly indirect; estradiol inhibits LH secretion by decreasing LH pulse amplitude and LH responsiveness to GnRH consistent with a pituitary site of action. Sex steroids seem to play a minor role in the feedback control of FSH secretion. On the other hand, inhibin B, the principal form of circulating inhibin in men, is the key factor involved in the testicular regulation of FSH secretion, as demonstrated by the inverse relationship between its circulating level and FSH ones.

Testicular factors

Testosterone is the main secretory product of the testis, the daily production rate being 5–7 mg in men. As the testicular content of testosterone in adult men is approximately 50 mg/testis, it is assumed that testosterone is continuously produced and released into the circulation. Testosterone is transported in plasma bound to albumin or to sex hormone binding globulin (SHBG), and only approximately 2% of total testosterone circulates freely in blood.

Testosterone plasma levels are strictly correlated to LH levels. Individual LH pulses in peripheral blood were found to precede testosterone pulses in the spermatic vein by 80 min, with a consequent strongly positive correlation among their levels in the spermatic vein. This correlation suggests the existence of a feed-forward relationship between LH and testosterone, which in turn reflects pituitary LH drive of testosterone secretion by gonadal Leydig cells. On the other hand, the increase in testosterone level leads to quite a prompt decrease in LH level (60 min delay) due to the feedback interplay within the GnRH–LH–testosterone axis.

Pulsatile LH concentrations bathing Leydig cells in the testes stimulate testosterone secretion in a dose-dependent manner. Some evidence suggests that LH and testosterone levels show circadian variations, with maximal hormone concentrations occurring during the later portion of night-time sleep. In general, the amplitude of LH pulses tends to vary inversely with event frequency and to be maximal at night, but mean daily serum LH and testosterone concentrations remain within a relatively narrow physiologic range, probably reflecting homeostatic feedback control. In young men, serum LH and testosterone concentrations are cross-correlated, reflecting LH's dose-dependent feed-forward action on Leydig cell testosterone biosynthesis as well as testosterone's negative feedback on GnRH–LH secretion. Reduction or removal of testosterone's negative feedback signal via an AR antagonist or an inhibitor of Leydig cell steroidogenesis increases the frequency and amplitude of pulsatile LH release. Conversely, continuous intravenous infusion of testosterone in steroidogenesis-inhibited men suppresses pulsatile LH release by reduced LH (and presumably GnRH) pulse frequency with escape of occasional higher-amplitude LH pulses [7].

Inhibin is a glycoprotein hormone secreted by Sertoli cells composed of an α-subunit disulfide-linked to one of two β-subunits, the βA-subunit to form inhibin A or the βB-subunit to form inhibin B. Its testicular origin was demonstrated when its levels were found to be undetectable in agonadal men and to be significantly lower than normal in men with other testicular disorders. Immunocytochemical investigation demonstrated the presence of inhibin α-subunit in both Sertoli cells and Leydig cells but not in the germ cells of adult human testes with normal or altered spermatogenesis. The βB-subunit was immunolocalized in pachytene spermatocytes to round spermatids as well as in Leydig cells but not in Sertoli cells in testes with normal spermatogenesis and with spermatogenic arrest. In testes with Sertoli cells only, the βB-subunit was localized only in Leydig cells. These findings suggest that germ cells could directly contribute to inhibin B production. In fact, it was observed that inhibin B concentrations fall to undetectable levels following loss of all germ cells in men after chemotherapy or radiotherapy. Moreover, a direct positive correlation between inhibin B and sperm concentration in healthy men is noted, and studies in which serum inhibin B levels were related to the histologic pattern of testicular biopsies have confirmed that inhibin B levels are reduced in men with severe spermatogenetic defects [8].

Secretion of inhibin B is controlled by many factors, including FSH and intrinsic factors involving Sertoli, Leydig, and germ cells. There are two discrete developmental periods in which there is a rise in FSH secretion leading to an increase in inhibin B levels. The first period of increased circulating levels of inhibin B occurs following the rise in gonadotropins seen during the first year of infancy. The further decline in gonadotropin levels accompanied by an increase in inhibin B suggests that maturation of a feedback inhibitory system occurs. Inhibin B decreases gradually to a nadir at 6–10 years of age then increases rapidly in early adolescence to reach a new plateau at 12–17 years. The second cycle of FSH secretion, followed by inhibin B secretion and suppression of FSH production, occurs with the onset of male puberty. At puberty, there is active mitotic division with spermatogonial maturation and accumulation of germ cells undergoing spermatogenesis leading to an increase in testicular size. During this period there is also a dramatic rise in FSH and LH and a sharp increase in the circulating levels of inhibin B. Before the initiation of puberty, the Sertoli cell is the predominant cell type within the seminiferous tubules, while germ cells prevail over the Sertoli cells in adult testes [9]. This scenario may be required for maintenance of inhibin B secretion and FSH suppression before puberty.

IGF-1 is also biosynthesized in the testis. Specific IGF-1 receptors are present in the testis and have been identified in Leydig cells, peritubular cells, and spermatocytes. LH stimulates IGF-1 secretion, which in turn stimulates the proliferation of Leydig cell precursors.

TGFβ may be involved in the paracrine control of testosterone secretion at Leydig cell level; in particular, LH may use the TGFβ system to end or reduce its own steroidogenic action.

Interleukin (IL)-1α is produced in the testis by Sertoli cells and may exert paracrine control of testosterone secretion by stimulating the expression of steroidogenic acute regulatory protein (StAR).

Growth hormone (GH) plays a role in gonadal steroidogenesis and gametogenesis exerting endocrine action either directly at gonadal sites or indirectly via IGF-1. In male subjects, congenital GH deficiency may result in a delay in the onset of puberty and has been associated with decreased sperm counts and motility, and reduced testicular size. In addition, GH influences Leydig cell steroidogenesis by increasing the expression of several genes that code for steroidogenic enzymes, including 3β-hydroxysteroid dehydrogenase, and by regulating the secretion of IGF-1.

Spermatogenesis

Spermatogenic cycles

Spermatogenesis is a complex cyclic process, where diploid germ cells undergo mitotic divisions, meiosis, and morphologic differentiation in a delicately regulated spatiotemporal fashion in the seminiferous epithelium (Table 1.2).

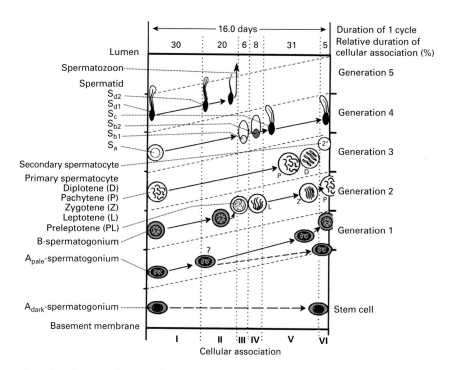

Figure 1.4 The cycle of the seminiferous epithelium. Examination of cross-sections of human testes reveal six cellular associations. The types of germ cells that should be present in each cellular association are illustrated in the six columns (upward from basement membrane to tubule lumen) as generations of progressively more differentiated cells. Relative duration (%) of each cellular association, on the basis of frequency of occurrence in specially prepared biopsy specimens from four men, is shown; coefficients of variation ranged from 18% for cellular associations I and V to 58% for association III. [Reproduced with permission from Aman RP. The cycle of the seminiferous epithelium in humans: a need to revisit? J *Androl* 2008. Copyright The American Society of Andrology].

The complex process of germ cell division and differentiation involves the completion of several stages (conventionally denoted by Roman numerals), whose number differs depending on the species. Rodent spermatogenesis encompasses 12–14 stages (I–XIV), while human spermatogenesis develops through only six stages (I–VI): the succession of stages through time is called the *spermatogenic cycle* (Figure 1.4). The spermatogenetic stages are precisely ordered: in rodents, stages that follow each other temporally are also spatially adjacent, so that the entire sequence can be described as a *spermatogenic wave*, while humans exhibit more than one stage per cross-section, due to a spiral arrangement of the spermatogenic wave. In humans, the entire cycle of six stages takes approximately 64–74 days; because differentiating spermatogonia divide every 16 days, there are usually four cohorts of maturing germ cells seen in any particular stage.

Table 1.2 Male germ cell types

Cell type	Ploidy	Cytology
A spermatogonium	Diploid (2n)	
B spermatogonium	Diploid (2n)	
Primary spermatocyte	Diploid (4n)	
Secondary spermatocyte	Haploid (2n)	
Spermatid	Haploid (1n)	
Spermatozoon	Haploid (1n)	

Human spermatogenesis can be divided in four sequential processes:
a. **Spermatogonial proliferation, differentiation, and their division to form preleptotene spermatocytes.**
b. **Meiosis of spermatocytes to preleptotene spermatocytes and second meiotic divisions to form spermatids.**
c. **Spermiogenesis, which is transformation of a round spermatid to a sperm-like mature spermatid.**
d. **Spermiation, which breaks structures and bonds anchoring a mature spermatid to a Sertoli cell, so the spermatozoon is released into the tubule lumen and can be washed out of the seminiferous tubule.**

a. Spermatogonia are diploid cells (2n) located on the basal membrane of the seminiferous tubule, which represent the precursors of all male germ cell types. Being the only germ cells that undergo meiosis, their function and integrity is crucial for the entire process of spermatogenesis. A continuous self-renewal process is then required, provided by stem cells that can undergo either mitosis (leading to daughter stem cells) or differentiate. Stem cells are a subgroup of type A spermatogonia that also comprise Ad (dark) spermatogonia (that may represent the reserve or non-proliferative spermatogonial population, which can give rise to Ap) and Ap (pale) spermatogonia (which are probably the precursors of B spermatogonia). Spermatogonia do not separate completely after meiosis due to incomplete cytokinesis and remain joined by intercellular bridges. These intercellular bridges persist throughout all stages of spermatogenesis and are thought to facilitate biochemical interactions allowing synchrony of germ cell maturation. Division of B spermatogonia leads to the development of preleptotene spermatocytes before the beginning of meiotic division.

b. Type B spermatogonia lose their contact with the basement membrane to form preleptotene primary spermatocytes (4n). Meiosis consists of a single step of DNA replication resulting in two chromatids per chromosome; during this stage, there is exchange of genetic material between homologous chromosomes derived from maternal and paternal sources. The exchange of genetic material involves DNA strand breakage and repair. The homolog pairs of chromosome migrate to a separate pole leading to secondary spermatocytes (meiosis I) containing a haploid number of chromosomes (2n), with each chromosome containing two chromatids. A second division (meiosis II) follows resulting in four spermatids, each containing a haploid number of chromosomes with a single chromatin each (1n).

c. Spermiogenesis (Figure 1.4) is the process by which spermatids acquire condensation and structural shaping of the nucleus, lose its cytoplasm and develop several organelles and accessory structures such as the acrosome and the flagellum. The nucleus is first located in a central position; as spermatids elongate, it moves to an eccentric position and undergoes significant condensation, reaching a final size one-tenth of its starting volume. This process involves the compaction of chromatin and replacement of histones with protamines, which improves DNA resistance to denaturation and leads to a decline in gene transcription. Spermatid cytoplasm is removed as a residual body containing remnants of the Golgi apparatus, ribosomes, some mitochondria, and is phagocytosed by Sertoli cells. Proacrosomal granules originate in the Golgi and form an acrosomal vesicle, which then flattens by incorporating newer vesicles supplied by the Golgi, spreads around the nuclear membrane, and when mature covering approximately 60% of its surface. The flagellum axial filament (axoneme) originates from the distal longitudinal centriole of the early spermatid and is composed by two central microtubules surrounded by a circular arrangement of nine microtubule doublets (2+9 system). The axoneme forms early in spermatogenesis and can be seen as a protrusion from elongating spermatids. The budding axoneme then lodges at the caudal pole of the nuclear membrane, leading to the formation of the neck. Periaxonemal components, the outer dense fibers, are assembled from small anlagen, and thicken throughout the remainder of

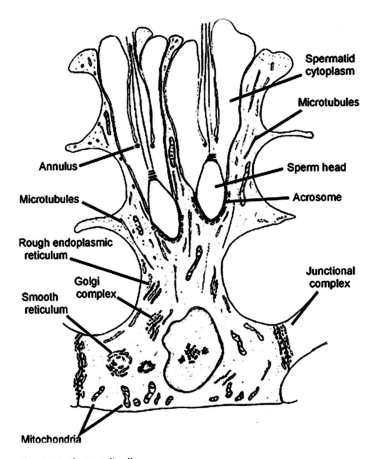

Figure 1.5 The Sertoli cell.

spermiogenesis. This assembly proceeds from distal to proximal, taking place through most of the spermiogenesis stages, and represents a crucial stage of spermiogenesis, as abnormalities of the axonemal structure are associated with some forms of male asthenozoospermia.

d. Once formed, spermatids are surrounded by processes of the Sertoli cell and reside close to the tubule lumen. As they elongate, their heads orient basally and become deeply embedded within the Sertoli cells, with their membrane tubu-lobulbar processes projected into the Sertoli cell cytoplasm. At spermiation, these attachments are lost and the spermatid is released as a free spermatozoon.

Role of Sertoli cells

Sertoli cells (Figure 1.5) provide support for developing germ cells within the seminiferous epithelium by participating directly in the deposition of extracellu-lar matrix components and permitting the formation of specialized cell junctions. Their cytoskeleton is responsible for the collective organization of the seminiferous epithelium and plays a crucial role in facilitating germ cell movement. Sertoli cells line the basement membrane and form tight junctions and adherent junctions with other Sertoli cells, which prevent the passage of proteins from the interstitial space into the lumens of the seminiferous tubules, thus establishing a "blood–testis barrier." Through extension of cytoplasmic processes, the Sertoli cells surround developing germ cells, provide an environment essential for germ cell differentiation, and are responsible for the movement of germ cells from the base of the tubule toward the lumen and for the release of mature sperm into the lumen. **The blood–testis barrier separates the epithelium into two compartments: the basal compartment, in which spermatogonia, preleptotene, and leptotene spermatocytes reside, and the adluminal compartment, in which meiotic spermatocytes and spermatids in various stages of spermatogenesis and spermiogenesis exist.**

Sertoli cells assist in the translocation of early meiotic spermatocytes from the basal to the adluminal compartment during the epithelial cycle in the seminiferous epithelium. This process, which likely requires the disassembly of Sertoli–Sertoli and Sertoli–germ cell adherens junctions, is a highly selective process [10]. Sertoli cells are indispensable to the release of mature spermatids from the seminiferous epithelium. This process involves a cascade of events, some of which include encapsulation of spermatid heads by Sertoli cell cytoplasmic processes, expulsion of spermatids from Sertoli cell crypts, and release of spermatid heads. After the release of mature spermatids from Sertoli cell cytoplasmic crypts, Sertoli cells phagocytose the residual bodies that were released from spermatids and any germ cells that may have degenerated during spermatogenesis. In this respect, Sertoli cells function as macrophages by maintaining the integrity of the seminiferous epithelium.

Sertoli cells also play an important secretory function: protease, protease inhibitors, hormone, energy substrates, growth factors, paracrine factors, and extracellular matrix components. Among others, the androgen-binding protein, a testicular analog to serum hormone-binding globulin, was first reported to play a crucial role in binding circulating testosterone in the testis. However, recent evidence argues against this. Sertoli cells are also involved in the transfer of nutritive products to germ cells.

For a more detailed description of this argument please refer to [2] (chapter 4) and [11].

Hormonal control of spermatogenesis

Based on the vast amount of existing data about this argument, there is only one thing that is certain: both FSH and LH are required for spermatogenesis. In spite of all researchers' effort, we cannot clearly circumscribe the individual effect of FSH and LH on germ cell maturation; therefore, the following assertions are open to further reappraisal.

FSH seems to be involved in increasing the number of Sertoli cells and spermatogonia, promoting spermatogonial maturation and enhancing the entry of these cells into meiosis, through its interaction with specific receptors on Sertoli cells. FSH is also essential for Leydig cell–Sertoli cell interaction: in mice lacking FSH receptor (FORKO), low testosterone levels are observed even after exogenous LH administration, suggesting a derangement in Leydig cell–Sertoli cell interaction due to absence of FSH signaling in the Sertoli cell. **In other words, FSH is required for the correct performance of the basal compartment of the seminiferous tubule. The employment of exogenous FSH treatment in oligoasthenozoospermic infertile patients has further suggested that FSH may play a role in the *qualitative control* of spermatogenesis, as** those patients achieve a significant improvement in sperm structure (DNA, acrosome, axoneme) after treatment.

LH exerts a crucial role in spermatogenesis, as it is required for testosterone biosynthesis. The principal effect of testosterone appears to be through increased entry into meiosis and, crucially, by enabling completion of meiosis. **Thus, the postmeiotic maturation is strictly androgen-dependent.** As a matter of fact, absence of AR, either ubiquitously through a mutation in the receptor (*Tfm*) or specifically in the Sertoli cells (SCARKO) will cause arrest of spermatogenesis in early meiosis. **Spermiogenesis is also testosterone-dependent**, as withdrawal of testosterone results in a premature detachment of round spermatids from the Sertoli cells leading to a marked lowering of elongated spermatid numbers. On the contrary, lack of FSH and/or FSH receptor does not affect spermiogenesis.

Steroidogenesis

Biosynthesis

Androgens are essential for spermatogenesis, maturation of secondary sexual characteristics, masculine settlement of the bone–muscle apparatus, and libido. Testosterone is the most important circulating androgen in men's blood. It is produced by Leydig cells, primarily in response to LH, which has both rapid (acute) and long-term (trophic) effects on their testosterone production. LH binds to specific high-affinity receptors on the Leydig cell plasma membrane, and the resulting accumulation in cAMP intracellular levels and the concomitant activation of the cAMP-dependent protein kinase A lead to phosphorylation of numerous proteins, including StAR. Steroid production in gonadal and adrenal cells requires both de novo synthesis and protein kinase A-dependent phosphorylation of StAR protein. The newly synthesized StAR is functional and plays a critical role in cholesterol transfer from the outer to the inner mitochondrial membrane.

LH stimulation is critical in regulating the rate-limiting conversion of cholesterol to pregnenolone within Leydig cell mitochondria by the cytochrome P-450 cholesterol side chain cleavage enzyme complex located on the inner mitochondrial membrane. This is a multienzymatic process, in which free cholesterol from

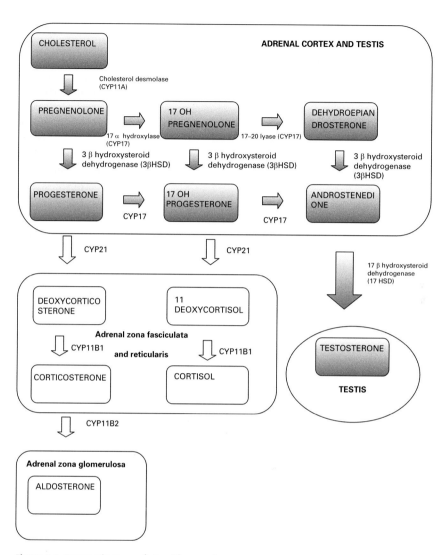

Figure 1.6 Enzymatic steps of steroidogenesis.

intracellular stores is transferred to the outer and then to the inner mitochondrial membrane. Inside mitochondria, cholesterol is converted to pregnenolone, a reaction catalyzed by the cholesterol desmolase enzyme (CYP11A). Pregnenolone is further metabolized to progesterone by mitochondrial or microsomal 3β-hydroxysteroid dehydrogenase. In Leydig cell smooth endoplasmic reticulum, maturation of progesterone to androstenedione is catalyzed by 17α-hydroxylase/C17–20 lyase (CYP17), whereas further conversion of androstenedione to testosterone depends on 17β-hydroxysteroid dehydrogenase activity (Figure 1.6).

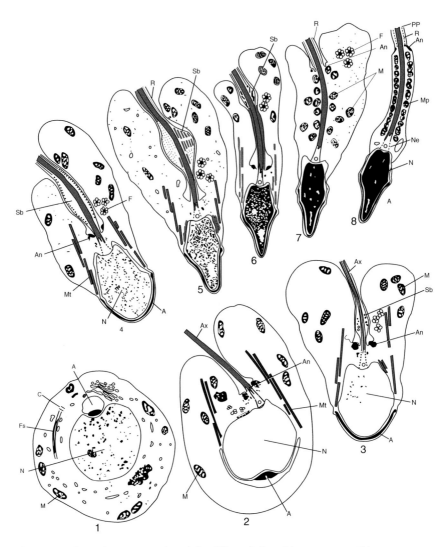

Figure 1.7 Schematic representation of the differentiation of human spermatide.
1, Golgi phase; 2–4, cap phase; 5–6, acrosome phase; 7–8, maturation phase; A, acrosome;
An, annulus; Ax, axoneme; C, centriole; F, flower-like structures; Fs, flagellar substructures;
M, mitochondria; Mp, middle piece; Mt, manchette; Ne, neck; N, nucleus; PP, principal
piece; R, ring fibers; Sb, spindle-shaped body. [Reproduced with permission from
Holdstein AF, Roosen-Runge EC 1981. *Atlas of Human Spermatogenesis*.
Grosse, Berlin.]

There may be also non-LH-dependent production of testosterone, which
was found to be critical in maintaining spermatogenesis under conditions of
LH inhibition; however, circulating testosterone levels are low under these
circumstances.

Secretion

Testosterone is secreted at adult levels during four periods of male life: transiently during the first trimester of intrauterine life, when masculine genital tract differentiation occurs; during early neonatal life; at puberty, when a remarkable increase in testosterone secretion is responsible for dramatic somatic changes; and continually after puberty to maintain virilization and spermatogenesis. After middle age, there are gradual decreases in circulating testosterone as well as increases in gonadotropin and SHBG levels, due to impaired hypothalamic regulation of testicular function, Leydig cell dysfunction, and atherosclerosis of testicular vessels.

Testosterone leaves the testis by diffusing down a concentration gradient across cell membranes into the bloodstream, with smaller amounts appearing in the lymphatics and tubule fluid. After puberty, over 95% of circulating testosterone is derived from testicular secretion with the remainder arising from extragonadal conversion of precursors originating from the adrenal cortex, which display low intrinsic androgenic potency. On the other hand, children's blood testosterone is derived approximately equally from direct gonadal secretion and indirectly from peripheral conversion of adrenal androgen.

Under normal physiologic conditions in young men, 4–6 mg of testosterone is secreted by the testes daily with a circadian rhythm; the highest level of secretion is in the early morning, and lower levels are found in the circulation during afternoon. This pattern is blunted with age, likely due to impairment at multiple levels of the hypothalamic–pituitary–testicular axis. A small percentage of testosterone (~1%) is converted to dihydrotestosterone within the testes and elsewhere by isoenzymes 5α-reductase I and II, resulting in circulating dihydrotestosterone levels in the 1–3 nmol/liter range in healthy men. Dihydrotestosterone is thought to be a considerably more potent androgen than testosterone due to its 10-fold greater affinity for AR, but its role in spermatogenesis is not known.

Transport

Testosterone circulates in blood by binding to circulating plasma proteins. The most important is SHBG, a high-affinity but low-capacity binding protein; under physiologic conditions, 30%–45% of circulating testosterone is SHBG bound, with the remainder bound to lower affinity, high-capacity binding proteins such as albumin and corticosteroid binding globulin, and 1%–2% remaining non-protein bound. Circulating SHBG concentrations are decreased or increased by supraphysiologic hormone concentrations of androgens/glucocorticoids and estrogens/thyroxine respectively. Other modifiers of circulating SHBG levels include upregulation by acute or chronic liver disease and androgen deficiency, and downregulation by obesity, protein-losing states, and genetic SHBG deficiency.

The clinical utility of partitioning circulating testosterone into derived fractions remains to be firmly established. The free (non-protein bound) testosterone fraction has been hypothesized to be the most biologically active form, with the loosely protein-bound testosterone constituting a less accessible but mobilizable fraction. However, the free and bioavailable testosterone fractions would also have enhanced access to sites of testosterone inactivation by degradative metabolism that terminate androgen action; therefore, these fractions may alternatively be considered the most evanescent and least active. Furthermore, empirical evidence indicates that, rather than being biologically inert, SHBG participates actively in cellular testosterone uptake via specific SHBG membrane receptors.

Mechanism of androgen action

Androgen action results from ligand binding to AR and translocation of the bound, dimerized receptor–ligand complex to the nucleus, where it directs androgen-regulated gene transcription via interaction with androgen response elements. AR is a member of the steroid hormone receptor family of genes, including receptors for steroid hormones, thyroid hormones, retinoic acid, 1,25 dihydroxy-vitamin D; the AR gene is located on chromosome Xq11–12. Like the other members of this family of transcription factors, the exons of the AR gene code for functionally distinct regions of the protein similar to the modular structure of other steroid hormone receptor genes. The first exon codes for the N-terminal domain, which is the transcriptional regulatory region of the protein. Exons 2 and 3 code for the central DNA-binding domain. Exons 4–8 code for the C-terminal ligand binding domain. The first exon contains several regions of repetitive DNA sequences: **a polyglutamine stretch, encoded by a polymorphic (CAG)nCAA – repeat, is present in the NH_2-terminal domain. Variation in length is observed in the normal population and has been suggested to be associated with a very mild modulation of AR activity. Either shorter or longer repeat lengths can result in a relevant biologic effect during a lifetime: shortening of the (CAG)nCAA repeat length was found to correlate with an earlier age of onset of prostate cancer, and a higher tumor grade and aggressiveness (but other epidemiologic studies in prostate cancer patients did not confirm this association), while longer (CAG)nCAA repeats may be associated with defective spermatogenesis.**

Upon entry of testosterone into the androgen target cell, binding occurs to AR either directly or after its conversion to 5α-dihydrotestosterone. Binding to the receptor is followed by dissociation of heat shock proteins in the cytoplasm, simultaneously accompanied by a conformational change of the receptor protein resulting in a transformation and translocation to the nucleus. Upon binding in the nucleus to specific DNA sequences, the receptor dimerizes with a second molecule and the homodimer entity recruits further additional proteins (e.g., coactivators, general transcription factors, RNA polymerase II) resulting in

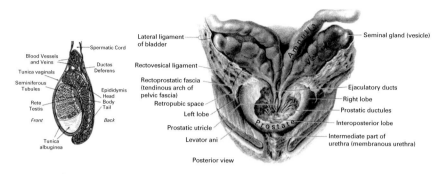

Figure 1.8 The male ductal system.

specific activation of transcription at discrete sites on the chromatin. AR is expressed in Sertoli, Leydig, peritubular myoid, and vascular smooth muscle cells, and on germ cells during the early stages of spermatogenesis.

The male reproductive ductal system

Epididymis

On the basis of histologic and ultrastructural differences, the epididymis can be grossly divided into three regions including the caput (head), corpus (body), and cauda (tail) epididymidis. **Each epididymal region carries out distinctive functions with the caput and corpus carrying out early and late sperm maturational events, respectively, while the cauda region primarily serves as a storage site for functionally mature spermatozoa.** The epididymis undergoes considerable remodeling, including duct elongation and convolution, so that by puberty the epididymis has acquired its fully differentiated state consisting of a highly tortuous tubule lined by epithelial cells. The development of a fully differentiated epithelium is dependent not only on androgens but also requires the influence of luminal factors from the testis (see Figures 1.7 and 1.8).

The adult epididymis consists of a pseudostratified epithelium of several cell types including principal, basal, clear, narrow, apical, and halo cells. The primary cell type throughout the tubule is the principal cell that constitutes ~80% of the epithelium and is responsible for the bulk of the proteins secreted into the lumen. Narrow, apical, and clear cells contain the vacuolar H^+-ATPase and secrete protons into the lumen and thus participate in its acidification, while clear cells are also endocytic cells and may be responsible for clearance of proteins from the epididymal lumen. Halo cells appear to be the primary immune cell in the epididymis, while apical cells may also endocytose luminal components. The principal cells also form tight junctions with one another and as such form the blood–epididymis barrier. This barrier creates an immunoprotective site within the epididymal lumen that is necessary for sperm maturation.

Several androgen-dependent transmembrane proteins, including occludin and claudins, contribute to the formation of these tight junctions.

The epididymal tubule is a highly ordered and segmented organ with each segment representing a unique physiologic compartment. Each compartment possesses distinctive gene expression profiles within the epithelium that dictate segment-specific secretion of proteins into luminal fluid directly or indirectly affecting sperm maturation. Segment-specific expression of genes encoding signaling molecules, regulatory proteins, transporters, and receptors also contribute to the formation of special microenvironments by allowing the epithelium to respond uniquely to different stimuli such as hormones and other regulatory factors. Despite this, the epididymal milieu should be considered as a whole, as perturbations in the microenvironment that surrounds the sperm cell could affect maturation. Indeed, alterations in luminal pH affect sperm maturation.

As spermatozoa migrate from the proximal to distal regions of the epididymis, they undergo a series of morphologic, biochemical, and physiologic changes with the end result being spermatozoa that have acquired the function of progressive motility and the ability to fertilize an ovum. Microscopic studies have demonstrated that, during epididymal transport, spermatozoa undergo remodeling that includes changes in the dimension and appearance of the acrosome and nucleus, in some species migration of the cytoplasmic droplet along the tail, as well as structural changes in intracellular organelles. The protein composition of the spermatozoon changes as the cells mature with some proteins disappearing, others being modified, and others changing their cellular localization. The biochemical alterations in sperm proteins reflect either those proteins that were synthesized during spermatogenesis or those secreted by the epididymal epithelial cells and interact with the maturing sperm. However, pregnancies were reported in patients with efferent duct–vas deferens anastomosis or with caput vasoepididyostomies, suggesting that spermatozoa may achieve functional maturity with either no or relatively little epididymal transit. However, it is believed that spermatozoa that bypass the epididymis have lower motility and fertilizing ability; by the way, the above-mentioned patients required up to 4 years to achieve pregnancy. Similarly, spermatozoa retrieved from the testis can fertilize oocytes in intracytoplasmic sperm injection cycles, but sperm motility and acrosome reaction are not essential for pregnancies to be achieved by that procedure.

Sperm movement through the epididymis is positive and pendular, as the fluid moves back and forth in the tubule. This movement establishes a potential for sperm mixing, as the cells make their way down the epididymal tubule. The propelling forces for sperm transport through the epididymis are hydrostatic pressure from fluid secretion in the testis and peristaltic contractions of the tubule. Sperm transit time through the epididymis takes about 2–6 days in humans.

A more detailed description of epididymis structure and function can be found in [2] (chapter 6) and [12].

Vas deferens

The vas deferens is an androgen-dependent organ that transports sperm into the pelvis, where it joins the seminal vesicles to form ejaculatory ducts, the largely collagenous tubes, which enter the prostatic urethra. Just before ejaculation, the testes are brought close to the abdomen and fluid is rapidly transported through the vas deferens to the ejaculatory duct and subsequently into the prostatic urethra. The vas deferens functions as a conduit between the epididymis and the ejaculatory duct. It is a tubular structure, approximately 35 cm, with a distinct muscular layer. It is divided into convoluted, straight, and ampullary portions. According to anatomical location, the vas deferens is divided into scrotal, inguinal, and retroperitoneal portions. Histologic examination of the vas deferens reveals adventitial, muscular, and mucosal layers. The muscular coat consists of inner and outer longitudinal fibers separated by a middle circular layer. During seminal emission, relaxation of the circular layer causes lengthening. Conversely, contraction of the longitudinal layer produces shortening of the vas deferens. The net effect of these actions produces anterograde propulsion of fluid. Contractions of the striated pelvic floor muscles subsequently expel seminal fluid during ejaculation. The pelvic plexus provides both adrenergic and cholinergic nerve innervations.

Ejaculatory ducts

There are two ejaculatory ducts, one on either side of the middle line. Each is formed by the union of the duct from the seminal vesicles with the vas deferens, and is about 2 cm long. They travel through the prostate and enter the urethra at the level of the verumontanum. The closure of the bladder neck sphincter prevents retrograde semen flow into the bladder during emission and ejaculation. Both the bladder neck and the urethra contain smooth muscle layers receiving a dual innervation from sympathetic and parasympathetic nerves.

Prostate and seminal vesicles

The anatomy and physiology of prostate and seminal vesicle function has been described in the 'Anatomy' section. The contribution of both glands in ejaculation is illustrated in the following section.

Ejaculation

Ejaculation is the final phase of the male sexual response cycle, representing a reflex involving sensory stimuli processed on cerebral and spinal levels, where a complex interplay between somatic, sympathetic, and parasympathetic pathways takes place. It consists of two phases: in the initial phase, *emission*, smooth muscles of the vas deferens, the seminal vesicles, and prostate, as well as their secretions, are involved. At the end, the mixture of spermatozoa from the epididymis and the vas deferens with secretions of the seminal vesicles, forming about 50% of the ejaculate, and the prostate, which secretes nearly the other half of the semen, is made available in the prostatic urethra. Sperm progression in the seminal tract during ejaculation and contractions of the epididymis are supported by oxytocin and guided by sympathetic and parasympathetic nerves. Neurons of the sympathetic nerves involved are located in the intermediolateral cell columns and the central grey of the spinal cord from T12 to L2, the fibers are part of the hypogastric nerves (in paraplegic men, stimulation of superior hypogastric plexus causes seminal emission). As transmitters, norepinephrine, acetylcholine, vasoactive intestinal peptide and nitric oxide have been identified. The parasympathetic neurons are located in the sacral portion of the intermediolateral cell columns (sacral parasympathetic nucleus). The emission process is influenced by central mechanisms via sensory stimuli from genital skin and from visual stimuli of the central mechanisms.

The emission is inevitably followed by the second phase of ejaculation, the *expulsion*, in which the ejaculate is expulsed through the external urethra, performed by a rhythmic contraction of striated perineal muscles. Expulsion is a spinal cord reflex that occurs as the ejaculatory process reaches a "point of no return." During the expulsion phase, smooth muscle fibers of the bladder neck contract to prevent semen flowing backward into the bladder, and the pelvic floor muscles (with bulbospongiosus and ischiocavernosus muscles playing primary roles) display stereotyped rhythmic contractions to propel semen distally throughout the bulbar and penile urethra. Although the bulbocavernosus and ischiocavernosus are striated muscles, their neurons share some similarities with autonomic muscles. They exhibit susceptibility to autonomic motor neuron disorders, they depend trophically on the presence of testosterone, and their dendritic arbors may cross the midline. Normal anterograde ejaculation also requires the external urinary sphincter to relax. The bladder neck and proximal part of urethra, both containing abundant smooth muscle fibers, receive a dual sympathetic and parasympathetic innervation. The external urethral sphincter and pelvic floor striated muscles are solely commanded by the somatic nervous system. The trigger of rhythmic pelvic striated muscles contractions responsible for the expulsion of sperm is still not clearly identified. It has been proposed that the expulsion phase of ejaculation is a reflex response to the presence of semen in the bulbous urethra. However, several lines of experimental and clinical evidence do not support this view in demonstrating that urethral stimulation by ejaculate does not contribute to the regulation of the striated muscle components of ejaculation.

An in-depth description of ejaculation can be found in [2] (chapter 9).

Brief excursion into sperm–egg interaction

Sperm–egg interaction is a specialized process that leads to fertilization. Once they have completed the capacitation, sperm cells bind to the zona pellucida. **This interaction is species-specific, requires the recognition between the two**

gametes, and evokes the acrosomal exocytosis. Acrosomal exocytosis is an irreversible process made possible by the presence of an intact acrosoma, which involves a complex series of intracellular events, resulting in fusion of the outer acrosomal membrane and overlying plasma membrane, with the subsequent release of the acrosomal content and exposure of the inner acrosomal membrane. The occurrence of acrosomal exocytosis facilitates sperm penetration through the zona pellucida, and exposure of certain molecules on the sperm equatorial segment that participate in fusion with the oolemma.

During penetration, spermatozoa beat their tails vigorously. It has yet to be ascertained whether spermatozoa would complete zona pellucida penetration solely by physical thrust (mechanical hypothesis) or requiring enzymatic activity without the contribution of motility (enzymatic hypothesis), or finally with the contribution of both mechanisms. It is noteworthy, however, that abnormal acrosin enzymatic activity has been associated with infertility and poorer in-vitro fertilization outcome.

Once zona pellucida penetration is completed, spermatozoa reach the perivitelline space and bind and fuse to the oolemma. This step is made possible by changes in sperm plasma membrane occurring after acrosomal exocytosis, and would involve the contact and binding between sperm receptors located in the acrosomal membrane and oolemma microvilli. Once spermatozoon has entered the ooplasm, the block of polyspermia is achieved by changes in the oolemma that prevent the entry of additional sperm cells (cortical reaction) and by enzymatic modifications of the zona pellucid glycoprotein, altering the structure and penetrability of zona pellucida matrix.

A more detailed description of a sperm–egg interaction can be found in [2] (chapter 7).

REFERENCES

[1] Zegers-Hochschild F, Adamson GD, de Mouzon J, *et al.* for ICMART and WHO. International Committee for Monitoring Assisted Reproductive Technology (ICMART) and the World Health Organization (WHO) revised glossary of ART terminology 2009. *Fertil Steril* 2009; **92**: 1520–4.

[2] Lipshultz L, Howards S, Niederberger C, eds. *Infertility in the Male*, 4th edn (Cambridge: Cambridge University Press, 2009).

[3] Hutson JM, Hasthorpe S, Heyns CF. Anatomical and functional aspects of testicular descent and cryptorchidism. *Endocr Rev* 1997; **18**: 259–80.

[4] Ascoli M, Fanelli F, Segaloff DL. The lutropin/choriogonadotropin receptor, a 2002 perspective. *Endocr Rev* 2002; **23**(2): 141–74.

[5] Padmanabhan V, Evans NP, Dahl GE, *et al.* Evidence for short or ultrashort loop negative feedback of gonadotropin-releasing hormone secretion. *Neuroendocrinology* 1995; **62**: 248–58.

[6] Bergendahl M, Evans WE, Veldhuis JD. Current concepts on ultradian rhythms of luteinizing hormone secretion in the human. *Hum Reprod Update* 1996; **2**: 507–18.

[7] Keenan D, Veldhuis JD. A biomathematical model of time-delayed feed-back in the human male hypothalamic-pituitary-Leydig cell axis. *Am J Physiol* 1998; **275**: E157–76.

[8] Marchetti C, Hamdane M, Mitchell V, *et al.* Immunolocalization of inhibin and activin α and βB subunits and expression of corresponding messenger RNAs in the human adult testis. *Biol Reprod* 2003; **68**: 230–5.

[9] Crofton PM, Evans AE, Groome NP, *et al.* Inhibin B in boys from birth to adulthood: relationship with age, pubertal stage, FSH and testosterone. *Clin Endocrinol* 2002; **56**: 215–21.

[10] Abel MH, Baker PJ, Charlton HM, *et al.* Spermatogenesis and Sertoli cell activity in mice lacking Sertoli cell receptors for follicle-stimulating hormone and androgen. *Endocrinology* 2008; **149**: 3279–85.

[11] Mruk DD, Cheng CY. Sertoli-Sertoli and Sertoli-germ cell interactions and their significance in germ cell movement in the seminiferous epithelium during spermatogenesis. *Endocr Rev* 2004; **25**: 747–806.

[12] Cornwall GA. New insights into epididymal biology and function. *Hum Reprod Update* 2009; **15**: 213–27.

2

Clinical evaluation of the male

Craig Niederberger, MD, FACS

Male infertility is extraordinarily common, contributing to approximately half of couples experiencing difficulty conceiving (see [1], p. 153). While their female partners are often communicative with friends and family about their reproductive disappointments, men usually are not, and it can be a great relief for a patient to understand that he is not the only man who is having difficulty impregnating his wife.

Why evaluate the male?

In the case of azoospermia, the only chance at getting sperm for the artificial reproductive techniques (described later in Chapter 8 of this book, e.g., in vitro fertilization [IVF] and intracytoplasmic sperm injection [ICSI]) lies in diagnosing the problem and, if necessary, harvesting sperm. When some sperm are already present but may be in low amounts or are of poor quality, the health of the man may be ignored in the rush to create a baby. To this end, IVF and ICSI have been both a blessing and a curse. These techniques are undeniably marvelous achievements that make life possible where it previously had no chance. However, they also allow the possibility of ignoring men in creating offspring.

So, why evaluate the man? In the first place, it is simply good medicine. Diagnosing pathology and treating it is what doctors do. Equally as important if not more so is that if you identify a problem amenable to therapy, you may lessen the intensity of artificial reproductive techniques required, perhaps rendering the couple able to conceive naturally. In the azoospermic man, your therapy may result in sperm in the ejaculate for IVF/ICSI, obviating the need for surgical retrieval of sperm from the testis. Therapy for the severely oligospermic

An Introduction to Male Reproductive Medicine, ed. Craig Niederberger. Published by Cambridge University Press. © Cambridge University Press 2011.

patient may result in enough sperm for intrauterine insemination (IUI) rather than the more costly and invasive IVF. For the oligospermic man, therapy may achieve sufficient sperm for intercourse to result in offspring. Finally, evaluating the infertile man may uncover comorbid diagnoses that left untreated would confer substantial harm to your patient. At least 1% of men presenting for infertility will have associated life-threatening diseases such as cancer [2].

Male reproductive history

How do we define infertility? Unlike many aspects of medicine where disease is identified by the patient as the discovery of symptoms, infertility is the recognition of something not happening. **For couples destined to conceive, each month the chance of becoming pregnant by intercourse is only about one in four to one in five, leading to approximately three of four couples conceiving after 6 months, and 9 of 10 by 1 year (see [1], p. 153).** It is important to communicate to the patient this probabilistic nature of infertility. Metaphors alluding to common games of chance can help, such as, "we're trying to decrease the number of sides of the dice so that the one marked 'baby' is more likely to come up." **The first question you will want to ask a couple coming for fertility care is, "How long have you been trying?"**

The second question to ask is "How old are you?" While recent evidence may suggest that the age of the father affects sperm DNA quality, without doubt the most impactful feature of any couple trying to have a baby is maternal age (see [1], p. 496). Nature is extraordinarily cruel to prospective mothers. By their mid thirties, when young couples are just beginning to get settled, female fecundity is on the decline. By her late thirties, a woman's chance of conceiving offspring faces a terrifically steep downward slope.

The third question is "Have you had children before?" It is important to know whether they have conceived as a couple, and individually with other partners in the past. Semen analysis might be an obvious test of reproductive potential, but having conceived and born a child is the most tangible confirmation that a man is able to impregnate a woman.

The remainder of history taking for the man who presents with concerns about his fertility is a combination of elements both standard and specific to male reproduction. You will usually ask about chronic illnesses, such as diabetes and cancer, past surgeries, medications, allergies, familial disease, and social habits.

Surgery involving the male reproductive tract can interfere with the passage of sperm. **Prostatectomy and "minimally invasive treatments" for benign prostatic hyperplasia often lead to retrograde ejaculation, and radical prostatectomy with its concomitant ligation of the vas deferens and removal of the seminal vesicles results in anejaculation.** Although the template approach to retroperitoneal lymph node dissection markedly reduced the possibility of anejaculation after this procedure for advanced testis cancer, the complication may still occur. Naturally, both blunt and penetrating trauma may incur damage to the testes and male reproductive tract. A pelvic crush injury may result in deranged anatomy obstructing the passage of sperm and seminal fluid.

An important surgery to inquire about is whether herniorrhaphy was performed. Mesh herniorrhaphy is associated with vasal occlusion [3].

History of spermatotoxicity

For the number of other, more specific pieces of information you will want to gather from your patient can be summarized in the mnemonic "TICS," as if you were ticking off items on a list. "T" stands for toxins, such as ingested chemicals. These may be medicines, both prescribed and over-the-counter, but may also be illicit, such as exogenous anabolic steroids or recreational drugs. A burgeoning category of potential toxins includes "nutraceuticals," or nutritional supplements commonly commercially available, but whose claims may not be subject to the same scrutiny as prescription medication. A more thorough list of prescription medications affecting male reproduction can be found in [1] (pp. 156–7), but common ones include cimetidine (which acts as an anti-androgen), alpha-blockers (which may diminish ejaculate volumes or cause retrograde ejaculation), calcium channel blockers (which may reversibly impair sperm fertilization potential), and chronic opioid narcotic use (which may result in hypogonadotropic hypogonadism) [1].

Marijuana and anabolic steroids may affect the male endocrine axis, with higher doses leading to lengthier and more profound effects. Your history should include how often and in what amount these substances are used. The effect of nicotine on sperm is controversial, but it clearly impairs penile function, and should be cautioned against. Caffeine neither helps nor hinders sperm, and as far as male reproduction goes, patients can be assured that they can drink as much coffee and tea as they like.

Cancer itself, particularly testis cancer, is often associated with decreased sperm production even before therapy is started. Chemotherapy, which arrests rapidly proliferating cells, also impairs the actively dividing and proliferating sperm progenitors in the testis. It is important to inquire about the duration of treatment, as longer courses of treatment are more likely to result in an irreversible halt in sperm production. **When chemotherapy is planned, I recommend offering sperm cryopreservation to the patient to preserve future fertility should the treatment render him permanently sterile.** Oncologists understandably want to rush therapy – after all, the man's life is at stake – but an afternoon spent freezing sperm may make a family possible in the future.

Like chemotherapy, radiation therapy directed at the testis impairs sperm production in a dose-dependent fashion. Typical times for sperm production to resume are shown in Table 2.1 [4]. Shielding the gonads does not necessarily prevent damage to the developing sperm. Patients understand that radiation damages DNA, and often inquire how long after radiation and chemotherapy is it "safe" for the sperm to impregnate an egg. At this point in medical history, we do not yet know. A recent thread on the male reproductive email user's group

Table 2.1 Typical recovery times for spermatogenesis after radiation

Radiation dose (rads)	Time until recovery of spermatogenesis
100–200	9–12 months
200–300	30 months
400–600	>5 years
>600	Permanent sterility

Androlog suggested that 2 years might be a reasonable amount of time for a man to wait should sperm return to the ejaculate [5].

As men evolved with their testes outside the abdominal cavity where they are significantly cooler than core body temperature, one form of toxicity is thermal. A varicocele is thought to exert its toxic effect primarily by raising the temperature around the testis. Likewise, if a man's testes are undescended, spermatogenesis is impaired, at least indirectly suggesting that the heat of the body is the cause. However, the underlying pathological mechanisms leading to aberrant germ cell migration might also be involved in the disturbance of sperm production associated with cryptorchidism. It is less clear what kinds of external application of heat, if any, lead to impaired sperm. A man crossing his legs, for example, raises his scrotal temperature by about 1°C. It is hard to imagine that men evolved so that the act of throwing one thigh over another quashed the chance of offspring. Similarly, laptops and tight underwear mildly increase scrotal temperature, but the actual reproductive effect of these elevations is not yet established. However, cooking the scrotum in the higher temperatures of Jacuzzi baths and saunas is more likely to lead to a temporary reduction in sperm production, and I typically counsel a man having a difficult time impregnating his wife to favor showers over hot baths during treatment. Finally, a febrile illness may temporarily mar spermatogenesis, and you will want to ask your patient if he's had a recent fever, and if so, when and how high.

Men may be exposed to toxins such as heavy metals in their workplaces, and asking your patient about his occupation and the chemicals with which he works can be revealing.

History of infectious disease

The "I" in "TICS" stands for infectious disease. Mumps may land in the testis, and if it does, a man is unlikely to forget the week both his cheeks and scrotum were painfully swollen. Urinary tract infections and sexually transmitted diseases may cause strictures in the lower urinary tract and epididymal obstruction. Although less common today, tuberculosis can cause strictures along the course of the vas deferens, leading to so-called "beaded vas." Controversy exists regarding whether prostatitis causes infertility, but if present, the white blood cells associated with the condition release toxic reactive oxygen species that may harm sperm.

Childhood history

"C" in "TICS" represents childhood illness. As previously mentioned, cryptorchidism is associated with derangement in spermatogenesis, with bilateral undescended testes exerting a greater effect than the unilateral form. The later orchidopexy is performed, the more spermatogenesis may be permanently impaired. You will want to ask your patient if his testes needed to be surgically repositioned into his scrotum, and if so, which side or both, and when. As discussed, if your patient experienced mumps in childhood, you'll want to know if his testes were affected.

Surgery on the bladder neck in childhood may also cause retrograde ejaculation, and hypospadias repair may have caused stricture, fistula, or may simply have been incomplete. External penile anatomy will be visible on physical exam, but internal anatomy will not, and knowing what kind of pediatric urological surgery was performed and when can inform you about how it may have impacted your patient's current interest in fertility. Because the vas is delicate and tiny in a small boy, herniorrhaphy may have unintentionally involved damaging it. Testicular torsion may have resulted in orchiectomy, or a twisted testis may have been untwisted after a time and then surgically fixed in the scrotum, leading to partial or complete necrosis. Asking about when a boy's voice changed, and when he developed facial, axillary, and genital hair, lends insight into whether puberty was delayed in the presence of an endocrine condition.

A chapter in this book is devoted entirely to genetics. **Common questions to ask of the family history are whether any blood relative had or has cystic fibrosis, or had difficulty impregnating or conceiving.** It can be surprising to a man having difficulty producing offspring that he may have inherited the problem, but genetics plays a large role in male infertility. (Please refer to Chapter 6.)

Sexual history

The "S" in "TICS" stands for sexual history. It is often surprising that couples frequently do not seem to understand that infrequent sexual activity results in a diminished likelihood of conception. Sperm is viable in the female reproductive system for about 2 days, and the window of opportunity for intercourse to result in conception appears to be 6 days before, and ending on, ovulation [6]. The problem is that tests such as basal body temperature and chemical assays reveal ovulation only after it has occurred. **Because frequent intercourse may dilute sperm counts if they are low, I recommend a target of intercourse every 2 days after menstruation ends.** It is important to emphasize to the couple that this schedule serves as a guideline. If, as many couples do, they rigidly conform to sex every other day and become greatly stressed when a day is missed or it accidentally occurs twice in a row, which is not helpful either.

Masturbation should also be considered as part of the equation in frequency of sexual activity. If a man has low sperm counts, frequent masturbation may further dilute the number. However, like intercourse, couples should understand that stringent rules should not be applied, and mandating a policy of no masturbation can be counter-productive.

The presence of erectile dysfunction is an important aspect of the sexual history. Men may suffer from the typical organic maintenance phase erectile dysfunction, suggesting underlying dyslipidemia and atherosclerosis that should be evaluated for overall health. In addition, the psychological stress associated with infertility, especially the need to produce sperm samples on demand in the reproductive endocrinologist's office, may engender difficulty in obtaining and maintaining an erection. A qualified psychologist with expertise in infertility and sexual dysfunction can be of great help to these patients. In addition, both organic and psychological causes of impotence may coexist, and often do.

It is important to ask about the use of lubricants during sexual activity. **Virtually all lubricants impair sperm, including saliva.** However, some couples need lubricants for intercourse. A recent survey of the effects of various lubricants on sperm motility and DNA quality suggested that Pre-Seed appears to have the least negative effect on sperm [7].

Finally, you will want to include in your history some basic facts about the female partner if you are not already evaluating her as her reproductive physician. Questions to ask the woman include assessment of anatomy, such as history of endometriosis, tubal obstruction, or pelvic inflammatory diseases, and overt symptoms of endocrinopathy, including irregular menses, and whether she requires medication for ovulation.

With so many aspects of the patient's history to discuss, if you're commonly seeing men seeking fertility treatment, you might want to use a history form that patients fill out in the waiting area or at home before seeing you for the first time. Our history form is shown in Figure 2.1. We also make it available on our website, so patients may complete it before their initial office visit.

The male physical exam

A good physical exam orients the physician to conditions for which the patient may be unaware. Nowhere is this truer than in reproductive medicine. Men may be missing a vas deferens, or both, and be understandably completely unsuspecting of this anatomic loss. Likewise, a patient may not realize that his testes are small. Men do not typically inspect each other's genitals. In fact, it seems that they are trained to look the other way.

A large part of examining the male reproductive system is putting your patient at ease. The first step is to act as if nothing is out of the ordinary. Should his partner be present, let the man choose whether or not she stays for the physical exam, and make it clear that it is his choice. Many patients will reveal

Male Fertility Questionnaire

Husband's Name: _____

Date of birth ____/____/_____   Social Security Nuber _____-_____-_____

Date of first visit ____/____/_____

Partner's Name: _____

Date of birth ____/____/_____   Social Security Nuber _____-_____-_____

Gynecologist Dr. _____

1. How long have you and your partner been trying to conceive with unprotected intercourse? _____ years _____ months		
2. Have you ever had a pregnancy with your current partner? If yes, how many pregnancies? How many went to term?	yes	no
3. Have you ever had a pregnancy with another partner? If yes, how many pregnancies? How many went to term?	yes	no
4. If yes to question 2 or 3, how many boys and how many girls, and how old are they?		
5. Has your current partner ever been pregnant with another partner? If yes, how many pregnancies? How many went to term?	yes	no
6. Have you ever taken Clomid? If yes, for how long?	yes	no
7. Have you ever had a varicocele operation? If yes, which side (*circle one*): right left both	yes	no
8. Have you had any other types of fertility treatments? If yes, explain briefly:	yes	no
9. Have you had a recent (within the past year) infection with a fever? If yes, when ____/____/_____ How high? _____°F	yes	no
10. Did you have mumps when you were a child?	yes	no
11. If yes to question 10, did it affect your testes?	yes	no
12. Have you ever been treated for a sexually transmitted disease? If yes, what disease? When? ____/____/_____	yes	no
13. Have you ever been diagnosed with tuberculosis? If yes, when? ____/____/_____	yes	no
14. At work, are you exposed to chemicals or pesticides? If yes, what chemicals?	yes	no
15. Have you ever been exposed to a large amount of radiation, or exposed for a long time?	yes	no
16. Have you ever had chemotherapy?	yes	no

Figure 2.1 A history form that the patient may fill out in the waiting area or before his visit.

		yes	no
17.	Do you take hot baths, saunas, or whirlpools? If yes, how often? When was the last time? ____/____/_____	yes	no
18.	When you were younger, did your testes have to be surgically brought into scrotum? If yes, how old were you?	yes	no
19.	Have you ever had a hernia operation? If yes, which side and when: right ____/____/_____ left ____/____/_____ both ____/____/_____	yes	no
20.	Did you ever have a bladder operation? If yes, what was done?	yes	no
21.	When you were younger, did your testes ever twist, requiring surgery to untwist them? If yes, which side and when: right ____/____/_____ left ____/____/_____ both ____/____/_____	yes	no
22.	Did you ever have major trauma to your testes? If yes, which side and when: right ____/____/_____ left ____/____/_____ both ____/____/_____	yes	no
23.	How old were you when puberty started?	yes	no
24.	Do you use lubricant(s) during intercourse?	yes	no
25.	Have you had any problems with erections?	yes	no
26.	How often do you have intercourse?	yes	no
27.	How often do you have any sexual activity?	yes	no
28.	Do you have diabetes?	yes	no
29.	Do you have high blood pressure?	yes	no
30.	Besides diabetes and high blood pressure, have you had or do you have any major medical illness(es)? If yes, what illness(es)?	yes	no
31.	Have you ever had any surgery besides a varicocele operation?	yes	no
	If yes, what and when?		
32.	Are you currently taking any medications on a regular basis? If yes, what medications, and what dose:	yes	no
33.	Are you allergic to any medications? If yes, what medications, and what happens if you take them?	yes	no
34.	Do any blood relatives have cystic fibrosis?	yes	no
35.	Have any blood relatives had difficulty to conceive children? If yes, which relatives (eg. Mother's uncle, etc.):	yes	no

Figure 2.1 (*cont.*)

	yes	no
36. Do you smoke cigarettes? If yes, how many packs a day? _____ For how long? ____ years ____months	yes	no
37. Did you stop smoking (*answer 'no' if you've never smoked*)? If yes, when? ____/____/_____ How many packs a day? For how long? ____ years ____months	yes	no
38. Have you ever used marijuana?	yes	no
39. Have you ever used any other recreational drugs?	yes	no
40. Have you ever used anabolic steroids or body-building drugs? If yes, which drugs?	yes	no
41. Do you drink alcoholic beverages? If yes, how many drinks (*beers, glasses of wine, tumblers, etc.*) a week? _____	yes	no
42. Has your current partner been diagnosed with an obstruction of her tubes?	yes	no
43. Does your current partner have (or had) endometriosis?	yes	no
44. Has your current partner ever had a serious gynecological infection?	yes	no
45. Has your current partner needed medication to stimulate her ovaries?	yes	no
46. Does your current partner have irregular menstrual cycles?	yes	no

Figure 2.1 (*cont.*)

information highly relevant to your diagnosis and course of therapy only after you are alone.

I leave some questions on the history to ask when I begin the physical exam, usually, "What kind of work do you do?" A man is typically comfortable discussing his occupation, and that comfort extends to the odd situation of exposing his genitalia to probing fingers. You will encounter the man who is uncomfortable no matter what, and occasionally on physical exam, your patient will have a vasovagal episode. Always be attuned to this possibility, aware of signs such as cool, clammy skin and sweating, and immediately have your patient sit should they occur.

With your first glance, assess your patient's overall body habitus. Although men with Klinefelter syndrome do not uniformly inhabit the tall, thin frame regularly described in textbooks, such an appearance serves as a clue that warrants karyotypic analysis. The presence of gynecomastia suggests an associated underlying endocrine or genetic condition. Likewise, scarcity of facial, axillary, or genital hair may be associated with endocrinopathy or a genetic disorder. Lack of closure of the epiphyses of the extremity bones results in abnormally long arms, and a larger ratio of lower body to upper body length as described in [1] (p. 200). The observation of this unusual body habitus suggests Leydig cell dysfunction before puberty.

Examining the testis

At the heart of the male reproductive physical examination is investigation of the scrotum and its contents. The scrotum itself may be hypoplastic on one or both sides, suggesting lack of contents since birth. The next component of the scrotal

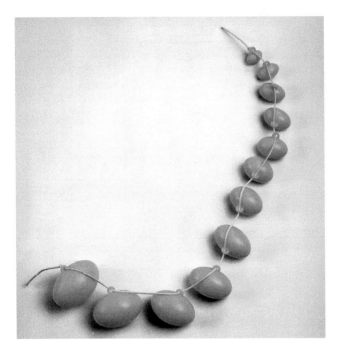

Figure 2.2 Prader-style orchidometer. Photograph courtesy of ASSI-Accurate Surgical & Scientific Instruments Corp.

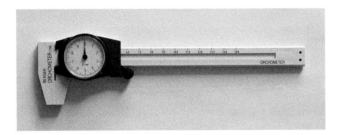

Figure 2.3 Seager orchidometer.

contents to evaluate is the testis. There are three commonly used methods to assess testis size. The Prader orchidometer consists of a string of oval beads with increasing volume. Figure 2.2 shows a Prader-style orchidometer. You simply try to recreate with the orchidometer what you palpate for the testis in the scrotum. **The typical threshold for the Prader orchidometer is 15 cm³, below that which is associated with substantial spermatogenic dysfunction.** The Seager orchidometer shown in Figure 2.3 is a plastic caliper that you use to measure the long axis of the ovoid that is the testicle. **For men with azoospermia, a testicular long axis of less than 4.6 cm strongly suggests spermatogenic dysfunction as opposed to obstruction as the cause** [8]. While Prader and Seager orchidometers are valuable tools in assessing testis size, the soft tissue between testis and skin render these methods necessarily inexact. For those seeking a more accurate measurement of testis size, ultrasound may be employed. Routine use of ultrasound in some centers has resulted in identification of subclinical areas of altered echogenicity in the testis, prompting the question of what to do with these lesions if found. At minimum, intratesticular lesions should be followed at regular intervals, and considered potentially cancerous, especially if found to grow.

The consistency of the testis is a key feature of the male reproductive physical exam. As the bulk of the testis' volume is comprised of developing germ cells, the testis is typically firm to palpation. Should the testis compress easily, spermatogenic depopulation is likely present. Small, soft testes in the presence of azoospermia make spermatogenic dysfunction the probable cause.

Immediately posterior to the testis, the epididymis can be palpated. The epididymis is a structure usually easily identified to be distinct from the surface of the testis, and is usually small and flat. If it is enlarged or asymmetric, epididymal obstruction or a spermatocele may be present. If only a portion is palpable, for example, the caput or caput and corpus, malformation from a congenital anomaly should be considered. In these cases, scrotal ultrasound is helpful in identifying pathology. It is important to note that no radiographic test can prove epididymal obstruction. That diagnosis is made by directly observing the epididymis during surgery, typically with the operating microscope.

If the scrotal sac is enlarged, a hydrocele may be present. In a darkened room, a light source such as a penlight illuminates the hydrocele. Hydroceles typically obscure intrascrotal anatomy, and ultrasound may be used to describe the anatomy within the scrotum.

Examining the spermatic cord

Examining the spermatic cord reveals two important structures, the pampiniform plexus of veins and vas deferens; both of which may be involved in male reproductive pathology. The varicocele is dilation of the veins within the pampiniform plexus, and is thought to disturb spermatogenesis by interrupting the countercurrent heat exchange mechanism formed by a central artery with blood traveling in one direction, and surrounding veins carrying blood in the opposite direction. In addition to the external location of the testis, this system keeps the developing sperm cooler than core body temperature, an absolute requirement for sperm production. The varicocele is discussed further in this book in Chapter 3. (See [1], chapter 18, pp. 331–61, for a full discussion of the varicocele.)

Many varicocele grading systems have been offered, but I prefer the simplest one, as it most directly corresponds to surgical outcomes. In this schema, a grade I varicocele cannot be detected on physical examination. Rather, the varicocele was observed only on radiographic evaluation such as ultrasound. This presentation is also referred to as a "subclinical" varicocele. **There is near universal agreement at this point that should a grade I varicocele be encountered in**

isolation, it should be left alone. (A subclinical varicocele in the presence of a contralateral clinical varicocele is still a source of controversy regarding whether to operate only on the clinically evident side, or on both.) This system is a variation of the original one proposed by Dubin and Amelar, in which a grade I varicocele is defined as one palpable only during Valsalva [9]. However, sufficient controversy around whether this type of varicocele should be treated calls into question the utility of describing a grade I varicocele in this way.

In the simplest grading system, a grade II varicocele can be palpated on physical examination, but is not visually evident. The traditional description of a varicocele on physical examination is that it resembles a "bag of worms," or an aggregation of convoluted subcutaneous veins that can be easily decompressed between examining fingers, squashing their liquid contents out from within. **Finally, a grade III varicocele can be visually observed by the examiner.** The veins are so large that their tortuous mass is visible beneath the scrotal skin.

The examining physician may use a pencil Doppler or duplex Doppler ultrasound imaging in cases where the spermatic cord musculature is so thick as to confuse identification of a varicocele. Using the pencil Doppler, the spermatic artery's auditory profile is distinctly different than the veins, with the artery making pulsatile short bursts, and veins sounding like the wind whistling through trees. With duplex Doppler ultrasound imaging, these structures can be visually identified, and the diameter of veins measured. A venous diameter of 3.6 mm or greater corresponds to a clinical varicocele, as does retrograde venous flow of greater than 1 second [10]. **Unless the physical examination is in question, I do not typically obtain Doppler studies, as a clinically evident varicocele warrants consideration of treatment, and a subclinical varicocele does not.**

You can usually find the vas deferens posterior and lateral to the spermatic cord – it is unmistakable. The vas is a firm cylinder and cannot be squashed like a vein, although do not squeeze too hard. The structure is highly innervated, and compressing it too vigorously will result in your patient feeling discomfort, typically in his lower abdomen.

One of the most difficult diagnoses to make is congenital absence of the vas deferens, as you are identifying that a structure does not exist. If you know how to do a vasectomy, you are lucky here, as you can use your skills in finding the vas deferens during that procedure to identify its absence on physical exam. **Try to pick up the vas in your fingers as if you were starting a vasectomy. If it disappears as you bring it up to the skin, and it keeps disappearing after two more tries, then it is not there.** This physical exam pearl is called "Meacham's maxim" after Randall Meacham, who described the technique. If you do not often perform vasectomies, diagnosis of an absent vas can be daunting, as structures in the spermatic cord can be confused by probing fingers with the vas deferens. Just remember that the vas is hard, and veins squishy.

The vas can be absent on one side or both, and each implies a different biological origin. Unilateral absence of the vas deferens may be due to lack of formation of the Wolffian system on that side, and the kidney may be absent as well. **If you feel a vas deferens on one side, but not the other, a radiographic** test such as ultrasound to investigate possible renal aplasia is indicated. If the vasa are absent on both sides, referred to as congenital absence of the vas deferens or "CBAVD," the etiology is related to the genetics of cystic fibrosis [11]. (Please refer to Chapter 6 in this book, and [1], pp. 262–4.) **If you find that the vasa are missing on both sides, cystic fibrosis genetic testing of both the patient and his partner are necessary to counsel the probability of having a child with overt cystic fibrosis should the couple consider testicular sperm extraction and ICSI for reproductive treatment. In 11% of men with CBAVD, a kidney is absent, so like unilateral vasal absence, a radiographic test such as ultrasound to investigate possible renal aplasia is indicated as well when both vasa are absent** [12].

Before you leave the spermatic cord, insert your finger into the external inguinal ring and inspect for the presence of a hernia.

Examining the phallus

The testes are where the sperm are made, and the phallus is where they leave. Hence, malformation of the meatus in hypospadias can result in semen being deposited too distal in the vaginal vault, or perhaps even not at all. If Peyronie's disease or other curvature of the penis is present, seminal deposition may be improper as well.

Examining the prostate and seminal vesicles

The prostate may be small, indicating inadequate androgen levels or congenital malformation. Likewise, the seminal vesicles are also expected to be hypoplastic in CBAVD and severe androgen deficiency, but these structures are not typically palpable on a normal physical examination. **In fact, if you can feel the seminal vesicles, they are most likely enlarged, suggesting possible ejaculatory ductal obstruction.**

Semen analysis

In this book, Chapter 7 is devoted to semen analysis, and intricacies of this important test are discussed there. This section describes the basics of interpreting semen analysis in the context of a man's initial evaluation presenting with concerns about fertility, or a couple who has not conceived within a reasonable period of time.

The bulk semen analysis is the oldest and most fundamental test of male reproductive potential. We call it the "bulk" assay, as it measures gross aspects of semen such as volume, and general population features of the aggregate of sperm cells, such as the concentration, and degree and quality of motion. However, the bulk nature of this assay is its primary limitation. Of the hundreds of millions of sperm typically ejaculated in a fertile man, only one will find its way into the ovum and fertilize it. **The bulk semen analysis does not directly identify the special swimmer that will ultimately result in conception.**

Another very important limitation of the bulk semen analysis is the great overlap between parameters of fertile men and those who are infertile. From MacLeod's original description of the semen analysis as a means of distinguishing fertile and infertile men, it was clear that they share a substantial number of similar semen analysis parameters [13]. One of MacLeod's solutions to this vexing problem of the relatively low capability of the bulk semen analysis to predict male fertility was to set the threshold for sperm concentration (also referred to as density, and typically measured in million sperm per milliliter), so low as to increase the accuracy in predicting whether a man is likely to have difficulty impregnating his partner [13]. The problem with this strategy is immediately evident, as a man may very well be infertile above this arbitrarily chosen threshold. The World Health Organization derived its set of parameters for assessing sperm from MacLeod's original work, originally setting 20 million/ml, and now recently 15 million/ml, as the cutoff value for sperm density [14, 15]. Unfortunately, many equate this threshold with normality, expecting that men with sperm density above this value are guaranteed fertile. **The only statement you can make about a threshold of 15 million/ml is if your patient's sperm density is below that value, he is likely to be infertile. You cannot assume he is fertile if his sperm concentration is greater than 15 million/ml, due to the substantial overlap between fertile and infertile histograms when plotting frequency versus sperm density.**

A more modern way of addressing the problem of when the affected and normal histograms overlap to a substantial degree is to create two thresholds rather than only one to define disease. Under the lower threshold, the doctor is relatively comfortable assigning the patient as afflicted, in this case designating the man as infertile. Above the higher threshold, the patient is more or less safely considered normal. Between the two thresholds lies an ambiguous "neverland," where the physician is unable to predict into which camp, diseased or normal, the patient under scrutiny falls. One modern statistical modeling technique that constructs just such a two-threshold system is "classification and regression tree analysis," also known by the acronym "CART." During MacLeod's time in the mid-twentieth century, the computational devices that allow fairly quick CART analyses were simply not available.

In 2001, Guzick and collaborators essentially recreated MacLeod's data, but calculated two thresholds with CART rather than one [16]. **Guzick and co-investigators found, for example, that at a sperm density less than 13.5 million/ml, a man was highly likely to be infertile, but above 48 million/ml, your patient is probably best assured the sperm concentration is consistent with unimpeded conception** [16].

A very significant limitation of the bulk semen analysis is its variability. Between samples, sperm concentrations may vary by the millions within a week, and over the course of a year, in the tens of millions [17]. One direct clinical implication of this great variability is that several semen analyses may be necessary before an adequate assessment of seminal character can be made. **Owing to the inconvenience that obtaining multiple semen analyses would place on a patient, our typical strategy is first to obtain two semen analyses.** If the two are widely divergent, then a third is performed. Occasionally, more are necessary, especially if long intervals have elapsed between specimens. The main idea to keep in mind is that as far as semen analysis goes, a single one is not enough.

Another profound implication of the sizable variability in semen analysis over time is the expectation that if a parameter is below the mean, it may rise on a future sample according to natural variation rather than responding to treatment. Any collection of measurements will have a number of them below the mean, and a number above. When sampled again, those below the mean will tend to increase, and those above the mean will tend to decrease. **This effect, called "regression to the mean," makes placebo controls essential when investigating medicines intended to improve semen analysis parameters.** All too often, studies record the same man's semen analysis before and after treatment, using the patient "as his own control." This practice is to be condemned, as if an initial semen analysis parameter was low, it can be expected to rise purely by the effect of regression to the mean. Only if a placebo control is present can the amount of improvement on a drug be compared with that of a placebo, and determined if the two are statistically different.

It is in the context of regression to the mean that WHO parameters for semen analysis can be most confusing. Whereas sperm concentration, for example, can be expected to have a mean value generally in the range of 100 million/ml, the WHO threshold for sperm concentration is 15 million/ml [14, 15, 18]. Thus, if a study included men with an average sperm concentration of, for example, 50 million/ml, it is expected that a future average density would be higher according to regression to the mean, even though the initial average was well above the WHO threshold for sperm concentration. **The important point to remember is that WHO thresholds for semen analysis parameters were chosen to maximize the likelihood of identifying infertility, not to specify normality.**

The most recent WHO semen analysis reference reports centiles for semen analysis parameters, and suggests a centile of 5% as the threshold for each [14, 15]. Men with parameter values above this threshold may certainly be infertile. By specifying a low threshold, the likelihood is high that a man is infertile with parameters below that level, but the converse (that he is likely fertile with parameters above that threshold) cannot be assumed. For descriptions of parameter values in the following sections, WHO thresholds refer to the 5th centile, as suggested in [14, 15].

Azoospermia

About the only truly definitive assessment of semen is whether sperm is present or not. The latter condition is referred to as "azoospermia," and must be verified by centrifuging the semen sample. Once azoospermia is established, the next diagnosis to make is whether it is due to obstruction, referred to as "obstructive azoospermia" (OA) or dysfunction in sperm production within the testis, referred to as "non-obstructive azoospermia" (NOA). The distinction is an important one to make, as in many cases OA may be resolved surgically, whereas NOA cannot.

Before the turn of the twenty-first century, it was necessary to perform a testis biopsy to establish whether azoospermia was due to an obstructive or non-obstructive etiology. This is no longer the case. OA can be reliably distinguished from NOA by two simple, readily available clinical parameters; a follicle-stimulating hormone (FSH) assay and testis size as measured by a Seager orchidometer [8]. **If the FSH is 7.6 IU/l or less and the testicular longitudinal axis is greater than 4.6 cm, your patient has a 96% likelihood of OA [8]. If the FSH is greater than 7.6 IU/l and the testicular longitudinal axis is 4.6 cm or less, the azoospermic man has an 89% chance of NOA as the cause [8].**

It is important to distinguish azoospermia from anejaculation. **Azoospermia is defined as the absence of sperm in the presence of an ejaculate, and anejaculation is the complete lack of an ejaculate. Lack of sperm due to absence of an ejaculate may also be referred to as "aspermia"** [14]. Azoospermia and anejaculation are entirely different. Azoospermia typically results from "upstream" pathology, such as sperm production disturbances in the testis or obstruction in the vas deferens, epididymis, and rete testes. Anejaculation usually results from "downstream" problems, such as dysfunction in the ejaculatory nerves, or obstruction of the seminal vesicles or ejaculatory ducts. Asking a patient with anejaculation if he experiences orgasm is important, as it can identify central nervous system involvement in his condition.

Semen character

Semen is ejaculated as a coagulum, and must first liquefy. This process begins a few minutes after ejaculation at room temperature, and is usually complete within 15 min [14]. Semen that does not liquefy within an hour should be considered abnormal [14]. To the naked eye, semen appears light gray and opalescent [14].

Semen volume

The WHO threshold for volume is 1.5 ml with a 95% confidence interval between 1.4 and 1.7 ml [14, 15]. **Practically speaking, it is not until volumes are 1.0 ml or less that clinical conditions manifesting as seminal hypovolemia become likely. These conditions include retrograde ejaculation, ejaculatory ductal obstruction, and hypoplasia of the prostate and seminal vesicles.** Hypoplasia of the prostate and seminal vesicles may result from congenital causes, such as CBAVD, or from profound androgen deficiency.

Post-ejaculatory urinalysis (PEU) reveals whether seminal hypovolemia is due to retrograde ejaculation. Post-ejaculatory urine is centrifuged and number of sperm is recorded. To a standard semen analysis laboratory, handling urine may be highly unusual, and you may find yourself explaining to a laboratory technician the necessity and technique of measuring sperm in urine. As urine volume may vary, sperm density is unimportant. Rather, it is the total number of sperm that is measured and reported for PEU. **The amount of sperm in the antegrade ejaculate determines the significance of the PEU sperm count.** A retrograde ejaculate containing 1 million sperm is highly significant if the antegrade ejaculate is azoospermic, whereas the same result in the face of 40 million sperm in the antegrade specimen is not.

Evaluating ejaculatory ductal obstruction (variably referred to in acronym form as "EDO" or "EJDO") is less standardized than retrograde ejaculation, and the diagnosis is consequently more ambiguous. **The most common method used to investigate the presence of ejaculatory ductal obstruction is transrectal ultrasonography, during which each seminal vesicle is measured in length and width, and the presence and size of an intraprostatic cyst is recorded, along with other anomalies such as intraprostatic calcifications.**

Jarow performed the initial anatomic work investigating the dimensions of the seminal vesicle, and it is on his statistical assessment that the ultrasound diagnosis for EDO is based [19]. **Jarow observed a normal maximum anteroposterior diameter of up to 1.5 cm for the seminal vesicles, and suggested that measurements above this threshold be consistent with a diagnosis of EDO** [19]. However, men with seminal vesicle diameters above 1.5 cm are not guaranteed to have EDO, and men with diameters below 1.5 cm may have EDO, a point that Jarow emphasizes. To more clearly specify the diagnosis of EDO, Jarow noted that the typical seminal vesicle does not contain sperm. **Jarow posits that if percutaneous aspiration of the seminal vesicles reveals numerous sperm, that result is diagnostic of EDO** [19].

Unfortunately, the easiest test used to diagnose EDO, ultrasound, is also the most ambiguous. Purohit and co-authors reported only a 52% concordance of transrectal ultrasound with radiographic assessment of seminal vesicles with injected contrast (vesiculography), only a 48% concordance with seminal vesicle aspiration, and only 36% of the time when dye was injected into the seminal vesicles, and cystoscopy was used to visualize whether or not the dye appeared at the ejaculatory ducts (also referred to as "chromotubation") [20]. In Purohit and co-investigator's study, approximately half of patients underwent resection of the ejaculatory ducts based on findings of these tests, and 10 of 12 showed some improvement in sperm count or symptoms [20].

With the lack of concordance between transrectal ultrasound, seminal vesiculography, seminal vesicle aspiration, and duct chromotubation calling the utility of each into question, Turek and colleagues have proposed evaluating seminal vesicles for obstruction with a functional assay, manometry [21]. Early results are promising, and we await larger trials with standardized thresholds to evaluate the efficacy of manometry in identifying candidates that would benefit from ejaculatory duct resection.

Sperm concentration

In the typical case, sperm concentration is reported as millions per milliliter (million/ml) and the WHO 5th centile threshold is 15 million/ml with a 95% confidence interval between 12 and 16 million/ml [14, 15]. This represents a significant departure from the previous WHO threshold value for concentrations of 20 million/ml, and it can be expected that many infertile men will have sperm concentrations above this value. **The Guzick *et al.* CART thresholds for sperm concentration were 13.5 million/ml and 48 million/ml** [16]. The implication is that if a man has a clinical condition such as a visible varicocele, but his sperm concentration is 28 million/ml, treatment is indicated. If, on the other hand, his sperm concentration is 80 million/ml, treatment is unlikely to substantially improve the odds for conception.

Sperm concentration is also called "sperm density." "Oligospermia" refers to low sperm counts, and "cryptozoospermia" to sperm counts so low as to be nearly azoospermic. If automated visual recognition systems are used to perform the semen analysis, it is imperative that a technician verifies cryptozoospermia, as debris may masquerade as sperm.

Total sperm number

Seminal volume multiplied by sperm concentration yields total sperm number, and is reported in millions. This parameter is valuable, as volume may be variable and concentration does not necessarily relate the total sperm available to impregnate. **For total sperm number, the WHO 5th centile threshold is 39 million with a 95% confidence interval between 33 and 46 million** [14, 15].

Sperm motility

Sperm motility may be difficult to assess, and is often inaccurately reported by labs infrequently performing semen analyses whose technicians may be unfamiliar with the appearance of sperm under the microscope. Everything moves at high power, and Brownian motion may be mistaken for motility, and vice versa. To complicate matters, several grading systems exist. The WHO 5th edition has a sensible and relevant grading system for motility [14]. Motility is divided into three grades. Progressive motility includes the percentage of sperm actively moving, either in a line or in a large circle, regardless of speed [14]. Non-progressive motility represents all other kinds of motility where sperm do not progress; for example, swimming in small circles [14]. Immotility describes no movement [14]. **The motility parameter typically reported for semen analysis describes progressive motility + non-progressive motility, and the current WHO 5th centile threshold is 40% with a 95% confidence interval between 38 and 42%** [14, 15]. This represents a significant departure from the 50% threshold of past WHO values. For progressive motility alone, the current WHO 5th centile threshold is 32%

with a 95% confidence interval between 31 and 34% [14, 15]. **The Guzick et al. CART thresholds for sperm motility were 32% and 63%** [16].

Total motile count

As semen volume, count, and motility may all vary, a good number to know is the total number of motile sperm ejaculated. This number is referred to as the "total motile count," and should be routinely calculated with every semen analysis. The current WHO manual does not list centile values for the total motile count, but it is reasonably calculated from the 5th centile levels for total sperm count (39 million) and motility (40%), yielding a value of 15.6 million.

Sperm vitality

The function of cellular processes within sperm is important, and is reported as "sperm vitality." **In order to assess vitality, sperm can be stained with eosin with or without nigrosin, and cells that exclude dye are counted as live** [14]. Those sperm that stain with the dye lack cellular processes to keep it outside, and are dead [14]. **Another method of assessing vitality is to immerse sperm in hypo-osmotic solution, the "hypo-osmotic swelling test"** [14]. Those sperm that swell are live, and those that do not are dead. This test is highly useful to choose sperm during IVF/ICSI, where staining sperm would prevent their use [22]. **For vitality, the WHO 5th centile threshold is 58% with a 95% confidence interval between 55 and 63%** [14, 15].

Sperm morphology

Sperm morphology can be one of the most frustrating parameters of semen analysis. Sperm shape is highly variable, and a normal man's ejaculate contains a broad assortment of strange-looking sperm. Until recently, two types of morphology were performed, a looser WHO morphology and strict morphology, but the most recent WHO manual abandoned the older method in favor of strict morphology [14]. Strict morphology is also referred to as "Kruger" morphology after Thinus Kruger, who invented the technique, and as "Tygerberg" morphology for his clinic [23].

Many methods of fixing sperm for strict morphology may be used, including Papanicolaou staining [14]. After fixation, sperm are inspected and measured, and if a sperm is identified with any abnormality, the whole sperm is counted as abnormal [14]. **For morphology, the WHO 5th centile threshold is 4% with a 95% confidence interval between 3 and 4%** [14, 15]. **The Guzick et al. CART thresholds for sperm concentration were 9% and 12% million/ml** [16]. The threefold difference between the Guzick et al. results, in which strict morphology was performed by a technician trained by Kruger, and the current WHO 5th centile threshold gives some indication of the strictness of current WHO parameters and moving nature of the sperm morphology target.

One problem with strict morphology is that technicians may be too generous in labeling a sperm as abnormal. You will find some labs that seem to report 0% strict morphology for every semen analysis. In those cases, it can be very useful to have the strict morphology assay performed by another lab that performs it commonly for comparison. I explain to patients that sperm morphology is like modern art: different people see different things in it.

If all sperm are morphologically abnormal in the same way, if they all have pin heads, or all giant spherical heads, then these represent genetic abnormalities with inevitable consequences for male reproductive potential. However, these conditions are rare. **One less rare but still uncommon uniform morphological abnormality is the case where all or most sperm have perfectly round heads, and are lacking the acrosome (i.e., the cap full of enzymes usually found at the tip of the sperm head).** Treatment for uniform acrosome deficiency is IVF/ICSI.

Commonly, you will see men in whom the only abnormality on history, physical exam, and semen analysis is isolated teratozoospermia, the term applied to aberrant sperm morphology. Keegan and colleagues studied men with isolated teratozoospermia undergoing IVF and ICSI, and observed no difference in outcomes in the first or second standard IVF cycle between couples whose men had isolated teratozoospermia and those with a normal semen analysis [24]. Further calling into question the meaning and utility of strict morphology when it presents as the sole abnormality in a semen analysis, Keegan and co-investigators found no improvement in outcomes when ICSI was used [24]. **Most men with isolated teratozoospermia who do not have other abnormalities on laboratory assay, notable conditions on history, and who have a normal physical examination can be reasonably assured that it is not the shape of their sperm that is the problem.**

pH and fructose

Fluid from seminal vesicles is alkaline, and that from prostate is acidic. Consequently, acidic semen may indicate aplasia or hypoplasia of seminal vesicles or obstruction. However, a hydroxide ion is terrifically smaller than a sperm head, and normal pH does not exclude obstruction. **The current WHO consensus value for pH is ≥7.2 [14, 15].**

Seminal vesicles secrete fluid rich in fructose, serving as an energy source for sperm. If fructose levels are low, aplasia or obstruction of the seminal vesicles may be present. However, like pH, a normal value for fructose does not exclude obstruction. **The current WHO consensus value for fructose is ≥13 μmol/ejaculate [14, 15].**

Leukocytes

White blood cells in semen indicate a possible infectious or inflammatory condition that may interfere with sperm function, and contribute free oxygen species harmful to sperm. (Please refer to Chapter 5.) **Under the microscope,** white blood cells may be confused with harmless immature germ cells, so staining is necessary to discriminate between the two. A capable technician can distinguish polymorphic neutrophils from immature germ cells on hematoxylin and eosin staining by the lobulated nucleus of the former, but stains for peroxidase activity such as ortho-toluidine can be used to more clearly identify polymorphic neutrophils [14]. The current WHO consensus value for leukocytes is less than 1 million/ml [14, 15].

Antisperm antibodies

Postmeiotic germ cells grow in an immune-privileged site, thanks to the barrier formed by Sertoli cell tight junctions. (Please refer to Chapter 5.) If this "blood–testis" barrier is broken, antibodies are formed against sperm. Conditions resulting in damage to the blood–testis barrier and antisperm antibody formation include testis trauma, toxicity, inflammation, infection and obstruction, as described more fully in Chapter 5. If a patient presents with low motility, particularly with sperm agglutination, and a history of one of these conditions, you will want to consider whether antisperm antibodies are involved.

IgG, IgA, and IgM are the salient immunoglobulins when it comes to assessing immunologic infertility, and it is their presence in semen and not in blood that matters. Although other techniques exist, the primary method to investigate these immunoglobulins in semen is to incubate with microscopic plastic beads coated with covalently bound rabbit antihuman immunoglobulins against the human immunoglobulins under scrutiny. This method is referred to as the "direct immunobead test" [14]. Sperm must be motile (typically with motility greater than 10%) in order for the direct immunobead test to work, as the technician observes the beads that the sperm drag around their head, midpiece, and tails, and reports the percentage of binding [14]. The current WHO consensus value for motile spermatozoa with bound beads is less than 50%, but it should be noted that the region where beads are bound is significant [14, 15]. Tail tip binding is far less important than binding at the sperm head.

Other tests

Numerous other tests exist for various aspects of sperm structure and function; these include how far sperm travels through cervical mucus, whether sperm penetrate hamster eggs stripped of zona pellucida, DNA fragmentation, and quantity of reactive oxygen species. These assays are not yet in common use.

Endocrine assays

As described in Chapter 1, the hormonal system plays a critical role in regulating sperm production, and endocrine assays yield important clues about the presence of conditions associated with male infertility. However, these tests do not take the place of a good history, physical exam, and semen analyses; rather, they complement and complete the evaluation of your infertile patient.

Assays of spermatogenesis

Currently, assays of spermatogenesis use the Sertoli cell as the "canary in the coal mine" of sperm production. The Sertoli cell is exquisitely sensitive to the germ cells in its folds, and inhibin B levels rise and fall with the number of developing sperm cells in the testis. **In its negative feedback loop with the pituitary, FSH levels indirectly reflect circulating inhibin B, with higher FSH implying worsening spermatogenesis.**

Inhibin B may be used to reflect sperm production, and some have argued that it is better correlated with testis size and semen analysis parameters, and therefore spermatogenesis, than the currently less expensive FSH assay [25]. However, FSH is highly correlated to testis volume and sperm parameters, and the benefit of using inhibin B as an assay of sperm production is incremental [25]. Today in my clinic, we use FSH.

As previously described, FSH level may be coupled with testis longitudinal axis to accurately distinguish azoospermia of obstructive origin from that of spermatogenic dysfunction. **The two numbers to remember are 7.6 IU/l for FSH and 4.6 cm for the testicular longitudinal axis.** If FSH is 7.6 IU/l or less and the testicular longitudinal axis is greater than 4.6 cm, the chance of obstruction is 96%. If FSH is greater than 7.6 IU/l and the testicular longitudinal axis is 4.6 cm or less, the probability that azoospermia is due to testicular dysfunction is 89% [8].

Before the era of microsurgical testicular sperm extraction with IVF/ICSI, men with FSH levels greater than two to three times the upper laboratory limit (typically 12 IU/l) were generally counseled to adopt. (See Chapter 3 for a description of surgical sperm extraction techniques.) However, Ramasamy and co-investigators observed that FSH levels, even high ones, do not predict microsurgical testicular sperm extraction outcomes [26]. **FSH levels can no longer be used to counsel patients that the likelihood of testicular sperm extraction is so poor that adoption is the only option if the couple desires children. The only reasonable use of FSH currently is to establish whether spermatogenic dysfunction is present.**

Assays of steroidogenesis

A critical component of spermatogenesis is the testosterone secreted by Leydig cells in the testis. **Although several thresholds for total testosterone have been proposed, the one most commonly used is 300 ng/dl** [27]. In the past, thresholds indexed for male age were employed, the so-called "age indexed testosterone," but this practice is to be condemned. It is similar to saying, the older a patient gets that we should accept a higher cholesterol test because dyslipidemia is more common in advanced age. When compared with any other illness, the capricious nature of an age index for testosterone becomes immediately apparent.

Testosterone circulates both free and bound to protein, and when the latter, either tightly to sex hormone binding globulin (SHBG) or loosely to proteins, predominantly albumin (see Chapter 1). **While there is some debate as to the activity of SHBG-bound testosterone, practically speaking, it is bio-available testosterone, free and loosely bound, that is of clinical relevance.** Currently, available assays for free testosterone are unfortunately not highly reliable. However, bioavailable testosterone may be easily calculated from total testosterone, albumin, and SHBG, which are all stable and reliable assays [28]. As of writing, an online calculator may be found at http://www.issam.ch/ freetesto.htm, and an application for iPhone, iPod touch, and iPad devices can be found at http://itunes.apple.com/us/app/bioavailable-testosterone/ id308770722.

Approximately 30%–45% of circulating testosterone is bound to SHBG in men, 0.5%–3% is unbound, and 50%–68% is bound to albumin [29]. **Thus, given a threshold of 300 ng/dl for total testosterone and assuming 2% unbound testosterone, bioavailable levels below 52% or 156 ng/dl, would be considered low, and levels above 70% or 210 ng/dl would be adequate.** Conditions that increase SHBG include hyperthyroidism, aging, hepatic dysfunction, anticonvulsant medication, and estrogens (see [1], p. 201). A decrease in SHBG may be found in hypothyroidism, acromegaly, obesity, Cushing syndrome, and exogenous androgens (see [1], p. 201). Whenever SHBG is well outside its typical range, a full endocrine evaluation, including a thyroid and cortisol panel, is reasonable.

As luteinizing hormone (LH) secreted by the pituitary stimulates Leydig cells to produce testosterone you can use the LH level to determine whether hypoandrogenism is due to pituitary or Leydig cell dysfunction. **A low LH implies that the pituitary is at fault, a high value implicates testis failure.** The distinction is important, as it determines potential therapy. If the LH is very high (e.g., greater than 25 IU/l), medical treatment aimed at stimulating Leydig cell steroidogenesis such as clomiphene citrate or exogenous human chorionic gonadotropin is unlikely to be effective.

If LH and FSH levels are near zero, the patient may have Kallman syndrome, a genetic condition caused by pituitary maldevelopment during embryogenesis (see Chapter 6). Other causes of pituitary dysfunction include tumors without or near the pituitary, and stroke. **However, androgen deficiency in the face of low normal LH levels is far more common** [30].

Testosterone is converted into estradiol by the enzyme aromatase. Excessive aromatase activity resulting in abundant estradiol may interfere with the male endocrine axis and sperm production. Raman and Schlegel use the testosterone (in ng/dl) to estradiol (in pg/ml) ratio to determine whether aromatase activity is too high [31]. **A testosterone to estradiol ratio less than 10 to 1 serves as the basis for aromatase inhibition therapy, such as anastrozole** [31].

Prolactin-secreting pituitary tumors may infrequently be involved in male infertility. However, symptoms such as visual field changes, headache, or erectile dysfunction usually accompany clinically significant prolactinomas. If such a symptom coexists with infertility, then it is reasonable to assay prolactin, but we usually do not obtain a prolactin level in the initial endocrine battery. The same is true of thyroid function tests. If SHBG is well outside the normal range, then we obtain a thyroid panel, but do not typically include thyroid tests among the initial screening ones.

If the prolactin level is high, repeat it before proceeding with an evaluation of brain anatomy, as prolactin is notoriously variable. The next step is typically cranial MRI. Mildly elevated prolactin levels in the range 20–50 μg/l are rarely associated with clinically significant tumors, and do not warrant further evaluation.

The initial endocrine evaluation

Based on the discussion in this section, a reasonable initial endocrine evaluation includes six tests. FSH indicates the degree of spermatogenic dysfunction, particularly in the evaluation for azoospermia. Testosterone, SHBG, and albumin are used to calculate bioavailable testosterone, with levels below 168 ng/dl arguing for possible hypoandrogenism. LH discriminates between the pituitary and testis as the cause for low testosterone if present. Finally, an estradiol level investigates the possibility of aromatase overactivity.

Genetic assays

Chapter 6 of this book is devoted to the genetics of male reproductive medicine, and genetic tests are not discussed in detail here. It may be very odd to patients to consider that the cause of their difficulty in conceiving children may be due to their genes, as they naturally wonder how it is that they came about in the first place.

Although the full human genome was sequenced in 2003, our understanding of genes and regulatory regions involved in sperm production is still lacking, and tests available to interrogate genetics are primitive. Two are in common use, the karyotype and the Y-chromosomal microdeletion assay. The karyotype may reveal numerical and structural chromosomal abnormalities. The Y-chromosomal microdeletion assay identifies a discrete number of regions on the Y chromosome that are missing. As the Y chromosome is the only one passed more or less fully intact from parent to offspring, if you detect that your patient has Y-chromosomal microdeletion, you can counsel your patient that if he has a son most likely the problem will be passed to his progeny. However, as the majority of genes by necessity go unscreened in current male reproductive evaluation, and much of male reproductive function is likely genetic in origin, you can counsel your patients that they may be passing "infertility genes" to their offspring.

The American Urological Association and American Society for Reproductive Medicine recommend obtaining a karyotype and Y-chromosomal

microdeletion assay for all patients who have a sperm density less than 5 million/ml [32, 33]. However, these tests are expensive, and the incidence of abnormalities varies widely by geographic region. If you find that where you practice, only a very few patients are identified by these tests, you may sensibly refrain from screening all men with low sperm counts.

Putting it all together

The male fertility evaluation is remarkable not only for its breadth – you will be synthesizing information from the history, physical exam, semen analysis, and laboratory assays – but also that it includes two patients, not just one. Keep in mind your patients' expectations and how much they want done. Some couples want everything possible in reproductive technology, and expect a baby as a result, while others desire first steps, and are uninterested in going further. **As maternal age is perhaps the most important predictor of reproductive success, how old the prospective mother is must be taken into account in the evaluation, and in how quickly it is performed.**

When assembling your history and laboratory assessment into a differential diagnosis, always remember a man usually has two testes. **A good testis producing sperm on one side may be blocked, and its opposite partner may be open but ailing.**

Azoospermia

Azoospermia represents an instance in which infertility is unequivocally related to the male partner. Figure 2.4 shows the algorithm for evaluating azoospermia. The first question to ask is whether the semen volume is very low. If it is, a genetic screen for cystic fibrosis should be obtained if either or both vasa are not palpable on physical examination. It is important also to obtain a cystic fibrosis screen simultaneously for the prospective mother, as the probability of cystic fibrosis in offspring can then be calculated. If the screen is negative, PEU is performed to investigate retrograde ejaculation, and transrectal ultrasound for ejaculatory ductal obstruction. If semen volume is adequate, FSH and testis longitudinal axis may be used as described earlier in this chapter to discern whether the testis is at fault, or obstructed. As described in Chapter 3, scrotal exploration for reconstruction is indicated for obstruction, and techniques such as microsurgical testicular sperm extraction are used to obtain sperm in men with azoospermia due to spermatogenic dysfunction.

Oligoasthenospermia

You will likely encounter low sperm counts and motility most frequently. It is important to calculate the total motile count, as that number will serve as the most reliable indicator of sperm production. It is also useful to explain to your

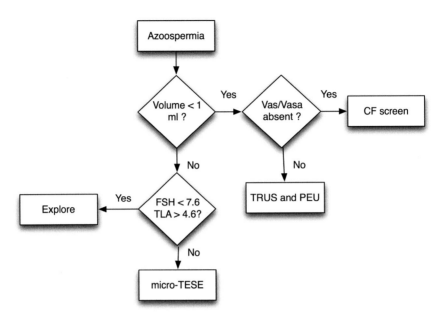

Figure 2.4 Azoospermia algorithm. CF, cystic fibrosis; FSH, follicle-stimulating hormone; PEU, post-ejaculatory urinalysis; TESE, testicular sperm extraction; TLA, testis longitudinal axis; TRUS, transrectal ultrasonography.

patient the natural variability in sperm production. Even though your treatment may improve sperm counts overall, the next semen analysis may be worse than the most recent.

Some conditions will correct without intervention, such as a recent febrile illness. Others, such as low testosterone or varicocele, will require treatment. **Always keep in mind, and communicate to your patient, what a reasonable expectation for the outcome of therapy is.** A patient with a moderate grade II varicocele and sperm count of 500,000 per ml is unlikely to achieve a spontaneous pregnancy with his partner a few months after varicocelectomy.

As discussed earlier in this chapter, when sperm are so few as to be difficult to count at all, it is referred to as "cryptozoospermia." In this case, it is important to explain to your patient that due to the variability of sperm counts, the next semen analysis may be azoospermic, but that does not mean worsening of his condition. The practical problem of relying on sperm when considering IVF/ICSI must be taken into account, however, when sperm may at any moment disappear.

Asthenospermia

If the count is abundant but the sperm are not moving at all, a vitality stain should be performed to exclude necrospermia. **If the sperm are live, one possibility is immotile cilia syndrome, where the structure of the sperm** axoneme is missing its microtubules or dynein arms connecting them (see [1], p. 179). If these ultrastructural abnormalities are coupled with other conditions such as situs inversus, the condition is known as Kartagener syndrome [1]. The definitive diagnosis is made with electron microscopy of sperm, which is not widely available. Another possibility for complete asthenospermia is antisperm antibodies, which can be a tricky diagnosis to make if all sperm are immobile. More often than not sperm are moving but motility is low. In this case, antisperm antibody testing may be revealing, as may pyospermia stain.

Teratozoospermia

With the advent of strict morphology and variability in what technicians call a normal-looking sperm, teratozoospermia has become a far more frequent finding on semen analysis. If it occurs with abnormalities of other semen parameters, then evaluation follows that of oligoasthenospermia, seeking the existence of other pathology, and treating it. If it is the only abnormal parameter, and all sperm are not morphologically abnormal in the same way, such as all having round or pin heads, then it is worth having another lab familiar with strict morphology repeat the assay.

Normozoospermia

With new WHO criteria emphasizing the 5th centile for semen analysis parameters, "normozoospermia" truly becomes the misnomer it always was. Once, values such as a threshold for density of 20 million/ml represented a consensus of experts in the field who proposed a practical limit of adequacy for a man impregnating his partner within a reasonable amount of time. The problem with drawing such a line in the sand is that it lulls the practitioner into thinking that anything above that number is normal. It is not.

Now, with the WHO 5th edition emphasizing the 5th centile as a threshold, the committee has sensibly stepped back from relying on opinion to set numbers, and instead performed a stringent scientific assessment of normative values for semen parameters. They could have set the 50th centile as the threshold (and the manual and accompanying journal article do report a range of binned centile values) but then plenty of fertile men would have been called infertile [14, 15]. Instead, the committee chose to pick a very low centile, the 5th, so that men below this threshold were likely to have a difficult time with fertility. However, men with parameters above WHO thresholds cannot be assumed to be normal, or even adequate. **The most important thing to remember when it comes to semen analysis, particularly when judged against the new WHO 5th edition criteria, is that if a clinical condition is present, it should be treated even if sperm parameters are somewhat greater than threshold values.** The whole notion of "normozoospermia" as sperm parameters greater than WHO thresholds is to be discarded.

Wrapping up

Fertility is an unusual field of medicine. Two patients are intimately involved, and the outcome is often like rolling dice. Evaluation can seem complex and intimidating, but if you approach it in a systematic way, with history, physical exam, semen analysis, and endocrine and genetic assays when appropriate, your evaluation will be complete and lay the groundwork for a rational plan of action.

Always remember you are part of a larger team, and work closely with the reproductive endocrinologist and embryologist teams to choose the best therapy. Keep in mind your patients' wishes, and manage their expectations; this medical field may seem complex to you, but to your patients much of it will sound like science fiction. About 99% of your job is to educate your patients what you would like to do and why, so that the whole team can make the most informed and sensible decisions possible. Communication is key; as you navigate the evaluation, keep everyone apprised of your findings and plans.

REFERENCES

[1] Lipshultz L, Howards S, Niederberger C, eds. *Infertility in the Male*, 4th edn (Cambridge: Cambridge University Press, 2009).

[2] Honig SC, Lipshultz LI, Jarow J. Significant medical pathology uncovered by a comprehensive male infertility evaluation. *Fertil Steril* 1994; **62**: 1028–34.

[3] Shin D, Lipshultz LI, Goldstein M, *et al.* Herniorrhaphy with polypropylene mesh causing inguinal vasal obstruction: a preventable cause of obstructive azoospermia. *Ann Surg* 2005; **241**: 553–8.

[4] Bahadur XY, Ralph YZ. Gonadal tissue cryopreservation in boys with paediatric cancers. *Hum Reprod* 1999; **14**: 11–17.

[5] http://godot.urol.uic.edu/androlog_archive/index.html

[6] Wilcox AJ, Weinberg CR, Baird DD. Timing of sexual intercourse in relation to ovulation. Effects on the probability of conception, survival of the pregnancy, and sex of the baby. *N Engl J Med* 1995; **333**: 1517–21.

[7] Agarwal A, Deepinder F, Cocuzza M, *et al.* Effect of vaginal lubricants on sperm motility and chromatin integrity: a prospective comparative study. *Fertil Steril* 2008; **89**: 375–9.

[8] Schoor RA, Elhanbly S, Niederberger CS, *et al.* The role of testicular biopsy in the modern management of male infertility. *J Urol* 2002; **167**: 197–200.

[9] Dubin L, Amelar RD. Varicocele size and results of varicocelectomy in selected subfertile men with varicocele. *Fertil Steril* 1970; **21**: 606–9.

[10] Eskew LA, Watson NE, Wolfman N, *et al.* Ultrasonographic diagnosis of varicoceles. *Fertil Steril* 1993; **60**: 693–7.

[11] Anguiano A, Oates RD, Amos JA, *et al.* Congenital bilateral absence of the vas deferens. A primarily genital form of cystic fibrosis. *JAMA* 1992; **267**: 1794–7.

[12] Schlegel PN, Shin D, Goldstein M. Urogenital anomalies in men with congenital absence of the vas deferens. *J Urol* 1996; **155**: 1644–8.

[13] MacLeod J. Semen quality in 1000 men of known fertility and in 800 cases of infertile marriage. *Fertil Steril* 1951; **2**: 115–39.

[14] World Health Organization. *WHO Laboratory Manual for the Examination and Processing of Human Semen* (Geneva: WHO Press, 2010).

[15] Cooper TG, Noonan E, von Eckardstein S, *et al*. World Health Organization reference values for human semen characteristics. *Hum Reprod Update* 2010; **16**: 231–45.

[16] Guzick DS, Overstreet JW, Factor-Litvak P, *et al*. Sperm morphology, motility, and concentration in fertile and infertile men. *N Engl J Med* 2001; **345**: 1388–93.

[17] Centola GM, Eberly S. Seasonal variations and age-related changes in human sperm count, motility, motion parameters, morphology, and white blood cell concentration. *Fertil Steril* 1999; **72**: 803–8.

[18] Fisch H, Goluboff ET, Olson JH, *et al*. Semen analyses in 1,283 men from the United States over a 25-year period: no decline in quality. *Fertil Steril* 1996; **65**: 1009–14.

[19] Jarow JP. Transrectal ultrasonography in the diagnosis and management of ejaculatory duct obstruction. *J Androl* 1996; **17**: 467–72.

[20] Purohit RS, Wu DS, Shinohara K, *et al*. A prospective comparison of 3 diagnostic methods to evaluate ejaculatory duct obstruction. *J Urol* 2004; **171**: 232–5.

[21] Eisenberg ML, Walsh TJ, Garcia MM, *et al*. Ejaculatory duct manometry in normal men and in patients with ejaculatory duct obstruction. *J Urol* 2008; **180**: 255–60.

[22] Sallam HN, Farrag A, Agameya AF, *et al*. The use of the modified hypo-osmotic swelling test for the selection of immotile testicular spermatozoa in patients treated with ICSI: a randomized controlled study. *Hum Reprod* 2005; **20**: 3435–40.

[23] Kruger TF, Acosta AA, Simmons KF, *et al*. New method of evaluating sperm morphology with predictive value for human in vitro fertilization. *Urology* 1987; **30**: 248–51.

[24] Keegan BR, Barton S, Sanchez X, *et al*. Isolated teratozoospermia does not affect in vitro fertilization outcome and is not an indication for intracytoplasmic sperm injection. *Fertil Steril* 2007; **88**: 1583–8.

[25] Kumanov P, Nandipati K, Tomova A, *et al*. Inhibin B is a better marker of spermatogenesis than other hormones in the evaluation of male factor infertility. *Fertil Steril* 2006; **86**: 332–8.

[26] Ramasamy R, Lin K, Gosden LV, *et al*. High serum FSH levels in men with nonobstructive azoospermia does not affect success of microdissection testicular sperm extraction. *Fertil Steril* 2009; **92**: 590–3.

[27] Wald M, Meacham RB, Ross LS, *et al*. Testosterone replacement therapy for older men. *J Androl* 2006; **27**: 126–32.

[28] Vermeulen A, Verdonck L, Kaufman JM. A critical evaluation of simple methods for the estimation of free testosterone in serum. *J Clin Endocrinol Metab* 1999; **84**: 3666–72.

[29] Bhasin S. Testicular disorders. In *Williams Textbook of Endocrinology*, 11th edn, Kronenberg HM, Melmed S, Polonsky KS, Reed Larsen P, eds (Philadelphia: W.B. Saunders Company, 2008) p. 647.

[30] Sussman EM, Chudnovsky A, Niederberger CS. Hormonal evaluation of the infertile male: has it evolved? *Urol Clin North Am* 2008; **35**: 147–55.

[31] Raman JD, Schlegel PN. Aromatase inhibitors for male infertility. *J Urol* 2002; **167**: 624–9.

[32] Jarow J, Sigman M, Kolettis PN, *et al*. *The Evaluation of the Azoospermic Male: AUA best practice statement, revised, 2010* (Linthicum, MD: American Urological Association Education and Research, Inc., 2010).

[33] The male infertility best practice policy committee of the American Urological Association and the practice committee of the American Society for Reproductive Medicine. Report on optimal evaluation of the infertile male. *Fertil Steril* 2006; **86**: S202–9.

3

An introduction to male reproductive surgery

Daniel H. Williams, IV, MD

The goal of this chapter is to introduce medical students, residents, fellows, and practicing urologists to surgical syndromes that can affect a man's reproductive potential. Descriptions of these conditions and their pathophysiology are accompanied by surgical techniques that can be offered to infertile men seeking treatment. The following topics and their treatments are presented: varicocele and varicocelectomy, obstructive azoospermia and microsurgical reconstruction, spermatogenic dysfunction and surgical sperm retrieval, ejaculatory duct obstruction (EDO) and transurethral resection of the ejaculatory duct, ejaculatory dysfunction, and electroejaculation (EEJ). Vasectomy is also discussed in this chapter. Imaging techniques such as transrectal and scrotal ultrasonography are described.

Varicocele and varicocelectomy

Varicocele refers to dilated and engorged spermatic veins that surround the testicle and the spermatic cord superior to the testicle. It is reported that roughly 15–20% of all men have a varicocele [1]. However, in the infertile population, varicoceles are found approximately 40–50% of the time [2].

Varicoceles are graded on a scale of 1–3. A grade 3 varicocele is one that can be seen through the scrotal skin without even physical examination (see [3] p. 343, figure 18.2). A grade 2 varicocele is one that is palpable on examination but not necessarily seen through the scrotal skin. Originally described as one that can be palpated on physical examination only with Valsalva maneuver, the modern definition of a grade 1 varicocele is typically one that can only be detected by radiographic assessment such as ultrasonography [4].

An Introduction to Male Reproductive Medicine, ed. Craig Niederberger. Published by Cambridge University Press. © Cambridge University Press 2011.

(a)

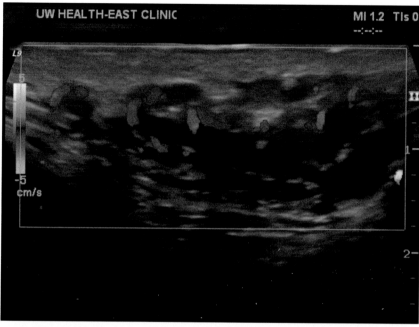

(b)

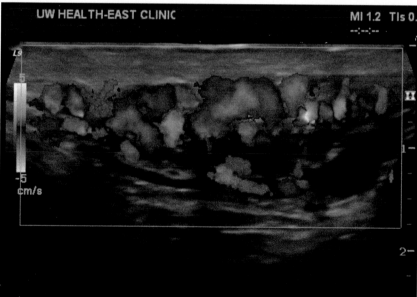

Figure 3.1 Duplex ultrasound of varicocele (a) at rest and (b) with Valsalva maneuver (see color plate section).

Scrotal ultrasonography (US) should be performed for varicocele detection only when physical examination is difficult or inconclusive (e.g., in a patient with thick or tight scrotal skin, or if the man is unable to tolerate the examination). The use of color-flow Doppler technology has allowed not only the precise measurement of the caliber of spermatic veins but also the presence of flow reversal with Valsalva maneuver [5] (see Figure 3.1).

While scrotal US is a valuable instrument in diagnosing varicocele, there are a few drawbacks to this technology. User experience and comfort level in performing such examinations varies from technician to technician. Additionally, radiologists interpreting the study results may use different criteria for what may be considered a clinically significant varicocele. Scrotal ultrasound is typically performed with patients in the supine position. In contrast, physical examinations are performed in the standing position when spermatic veins are most engorged. Patients with palpable varicoceles in the standing position should also be examined when supine to ensure that the veins deflate in this position. **Varicoceles that do not deflate when patients are supine, as well as isolated right-sided varicoceles, should raise the clinical suspicion of an intra-abdominal process and should be further evaluated with abdominal imaging.**

The exact mechanism of the deleterious effects of varicocele on sperm production remains to be elucidated, but a number of theories have been proposed. **The most widely accepted theory of how varicocele affects testicular function is that of elevated testicular temperature** [6]. It has been demonstrated that scrotal temperature decreases following varicocele repair [7]. Other theories include a pressure effect of a varicocele on venous return, oxygen deprivation, reflux of toxic metabolites from the kidney down to the testes, and impaired clearance of metabolites from the testes (see [3], pp. 332–6). Lastly, it is important to keep in mind that a unilateral varicocele can have a bilateral effect on the testes (8).

Regarding the surgical management of a varicocele, there are a number of approaches including retroperitoneal, inguinal, subinguinal, and laparoscopic (see [3], p. 343, figure 18.2). Radiographic embolization is another option to treat a varicocele (see [3], p. 345, figure 18.7; and p. 388, figure 20.25). **All of these approaches have unique advantages and disadvantages, including cost, recovery time, access to technologies and resources, and surgical skill.** Ultimately, the choice of management is up to the patient and his urologist based on these factors.

The most common approach to varicocelectomy taken by most male infertility specialists in North America is that of either an inguinal or a subinguinal microsurgical approach. Depending on the patient's body habits, either approach can be performed through a relatively small 3–4-cm incision. **Use of the operating microscope has been repeatedly demonstrated to not only improve surgical outcomes but also minimize potential postoperative complications such as hydrocele, testicular atrophy, and recurrence** [8] (see Figure 3.2). Using an operating microscope allows for easier identification of arteries and veins, particularly the small periarterial veins as well as identification of lymphatics. An operating microscope may also be connected to a digital camera, which allows added benefit of an excellent teaching instrument.

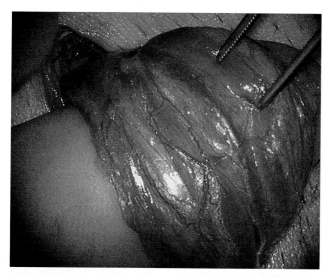

Figure 3.2 Spermatic cord structures as seen through an operating microscope (8×). From left to right: lymphatic (shiny, clear), vas deferens (white), vein (blue), testicular artery (dark red), vein (blue, under tips of forceps), vein (blue, behind forceps) (see color plate section).

When using a microsurgical approach to varicocelectomy, a critical instrument in the operating room is the microsurgical Doppler ultrasound probe. This is not a "pencil Doppler," rather it is one with a fine, 1-mm tip. Use of this device allows for meticulous identification of vital structures in the spermatic cord and results in the safest and most effective approach to microsurgical varicocelectomy.

Once the spermatic cord is delivered into the operative field, the operating microscope allows for easy identification of the spermatic cord structures. Depending on a subinguinal or inguinal approach, there may be either one main spermatic artery or multiple branches of the spermatic artery. **Sometimes large cremasteric vessels are present that also need to be identified and ligated.** Veins may be occluded with either hemoclips or non-absorbable sutures based on the preference of the microsurgeon.

The closer the incision is made to the testes, the more veins there are to ligate. For example, with an inguinal approach, there typically is one large lateral vein with one prominent testicular artery flanked by two smaller periarterial veins. When a subinguinal approach is used, it is easier to deliver the spermatic cord. However, there may be up to three or four branches of the spermatic artery, accompanied by their periarterial veins, all of which need to be ligated. **It is critical that all visible spermatic veins are ligated to ensure the best possible outcome.** Without using the operating microscope and microsurgical Doppler ultrasound, small periarterial veins may be missed, which can lead to recurrence.

Microsurgical varicocelectomy is a relatively quick (60–90 minute) outpatient procedure. Most men are able to gradually increase their activity level and return to routine activities within a few weeks. Microsurgical repair of varicoceles offers a lower risk of hydrocele formation, as well as lower risk of varicocele recurrence when compared with approaches that do not use optical magnification. **Semen parameters improve approximately 70–80% of the time, and there can be improvements in functional sperm defects** (see [3], pp. 347–54). For example, following varicocelectomy there is an increase in live birth rates with intrauterine inseminations (IUI) even without a significant change in semen analysis. This suggests an improved functional factor not measured on routine semen analysis that improves following microsurgical varicocelectomy [9]. Additionally, the World Health Organization has concluded that varicoceles are clearly associated with impairment of testicular function and infertility [10].

For men who do not desire surgical repair of symptomatic varicoceles, who have had extensive previous inguinal surgery, or in whom previous attempts at varicocelectomy have resulted in recurrence, percutaneous embolization may be offered. Occlusive balloons, coils, and sclerotherapy are all techniques that have unique advantages and disadvantages [11, 12]. Coil or balloon migration, exposure to radiation, and higher reported rates of recurrence are a few reasons why embolization is not generally recommended as a first-line treatment for infertile men with symptomatic varicoceles. Please see [3] (pp. 331–56) for more detailed discussions of varicocele and management.

Obstructive azoospermia

Obstructive azoospermia refers to no sperm in the semen of a man who otherwise has normal physical examination findings, including normal-sized testis, palpable vas deferens, absence of varicocele, normal hormone profiles, and nothing in his medical history that would result in impaired spermatogenesis (i.e., recent chemotherapy, radiation therapy, etc.). **Obstruction of sperm and semen in such cases can occur anywhere in the reproductive tract: at the level of the epididymis, vas deferens, or ejaculatory duct.** Diagnostic studies that can help pinpoint the level of obstruction include checking semen for pH and fructose, transrectal US, seminal vesicle aspiration, and ultimately scrotal exploration with vasography.

When obstructive azoospermia is present, sperm production by the testis remains normal and often epididymal tubules become quite dilated. The yield of sperm from the epididymis is logarithmically higher than the yield of sperm from the testis; therefore, in such cases where microsurgical reconstruction is not possible and sperm retrieval techniques are employed, epididymal sperm is often preferred. Epididymal sperm may be obtained through either blind percutaneous approaches or more meticulous microscopic epididymal sperm aspiration techniques (see Figure 3.3). Factors to consider for selecting each approach include patient's preference, cost, surgeon's experience and comfort level with the various approaches, and ultimate goal of the sperm retrieval (i.e., whether sperm will be used fresh for a single cycle of in vitro fertilization [IVF] with intracytoplasmic sperm injection [ICSI], or if the sperm are to be frozen for multiple potential

(a)

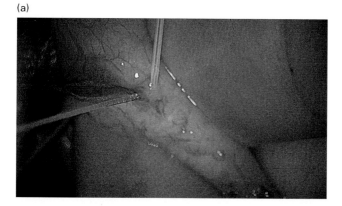

(b)

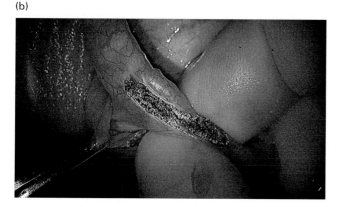

Figure 3.3 Microsurgical epididymal sperm aspiration (MESA). (a) An ophthalmological blade is used to open the delicate epididymal tubules while fluid is aspirated into an angiocath-tipped syringe. (b) Appearance of epididymis upon completion of an "obliterative" MESA (see color plate section).

future cycles). **In contrast to non-obstructive azoospermia (NOA), when sperm from a man with obstructive azoospermia are used for IVF/ICSI, success rates generally are excellent.** Please see [3] (pp. 409–12) for further information regarding surgical approaches to epididymal sperm retrieval for treatment of obstructive azoospermia.

Congenital bilateral absence of the vas deferens

In the setting of congenital bilateral absence of the vas deferens (CBAVD), which is associated with abnormalities of cystic fibrosis transmembrane conductance regulator (*CFTR*) genes, testicular production of sperm typically is normal (see [3], pp. 262–4). Sperm can be surgically retrieved from either the epididymis or testis. Once obtained, this sperm must be used in conjunction with IVF/ICSI.

If the vas deferens are palpable bilaterally, and if obstructive azoospermia is suspected, obstruction may occur distally at the level of the ejaculatory duct, or a blind-ending vas deferens may be found in the pelvis. **Men may also have obstructive azoospermia at the level of the epididymis, for example, following episodes of epididymitis, testicular injury, or in conjunction with CFTR abnormalities.** Microsurgical epididymovasostomy may be attempted in this setting (see below).

Some men may be found to have congenital unilateral absence of the vas deferens. **Unlike CBAVD, this entity generally is not associated with CFTR gene abnormalities.** Rather, it is thought that abnormal mesonephric duct differentiation occurring early in embryogenesis results in this phenomenon. Because the developing metanephric blastema may also be affected, ipsilateral renal agenesis may be present. Therefore, renal ultrasound generally is recommended when a man is found to have a unilateral absent vas deferens.

Ejaculatory duct obstruction

The anatomy of the male reproductive tract is such that sperm exit the testes, travel through the epididymis, and enter the vas deferens. The vas deferens travels into the inguinal canal with the spermatic cord and then dives posteromedially to fuse with the seminal vesicles at the ampulla of the vas deferens. Here, the seminal vesicles empty into the ejaculatory duct of the prostate.

Situations exist where the ejaculatory duct may be obstructed, either completely or partially. Complete EDO results in a total blockage of semen emission from the seminal vesicles. Partial EDO arises from anatomical situations where semen and sperm cannot be ejaculated efficiently. **The diagnosis of complete EDO can be made on semen analysis by seeing low-volume azoospermia with low pH and absent fructose.** Generally, men with EDO are diagnosed during evaluation of their infertility, as they are otherwise asymptomatic.

EDO diagnosis can also be further elucidated by transrectal ultrasound. **Transrectal ultrasound is useful in evaluating the presence and size of seminal vesicles and any ejaculatory duct cysts or Müllerian duct remnants that might be suggestive of EDO** (see [3], p. 380, figure 20.8). Although there is no specific thickness of the seminal vesicles that is pathognomonic for EDO, some authors report 15 mm as a thickness that should raise the suspicion for EDO [13].

Another procedure that can help diagnose EDO is seminal vesicle aspiration. This procedure is performed using a transrectal ultrasound-guided needle passed into the seminal vesicle in a similar approach to that of prostate biopsy. Once the needle has passed into the seminal vesicle, a small amount of fluid can be aspirated into a syringe and examined under light microscopy [14]. **Similar to transrectal ultrasound measurements of the seminal vesicles, there is no specific amount of sperm in the seminal vesicles that is pathognomonic for either complete or partial EDO; however, some authors advocate that more than three sperm per high-powered field is consistent with EDO** [15]. Before performing seminal vesicle aspiration, it is important that the patient undergoes preoperative preparation that is similar to prostate biopsy, and that ejaculation is performed within 24 hours.

If clinical suspicion for EDO is high then transurethral resection of the ejaculatory duct (TURED) may be offered. The approach is similar to that of transurethral resection of the prostate (TURP). However, rather than sparing the verumontanum and ejaculatory duct (which is often the case in TURP), the verumontanum needs to be resected in order to remove the EDO (see [3], p. 425, figure 23.5). Another important difference between TURED and TURP is that TURED typically is performed on younger men of reproductive age with small prostates. **Thus, care needs to be taken when performing a TURED not to injure the external sphincter or carry the resection too deep and damage the rectal mucosa.**

A very useful technique with TURED is chromopertubation of the seminal vesicles with either indigo carmine or methylene blue. After seminal vesicle aspiration is performed to confirm the presence of sperm in seminal vesicles, the needle can be kept in place and diluted indigo carmine or methylene blue can be injected. **Filling seminal vesicles with dye helps determine the limit of resection during TURED when the dye is seen effluxing from the resection bed.** A Foley catheter is then placed for approximately 24 hours, and early ejaculation following the procedure is encouraged to reduce the risk of scarring of the freshly resected ejaculatory ducts. Results of TURED include improvement in sperm concentration and motility in approximately 65% of patients, increased ejaculatory volume in about 30% of patients, and roughly 30% of patients will initiate a pregnancy [16]. Please see [3] (pp. 425–7) for detailed discussion of TURED and outcomes.

Vasal occlusion

Obstructive azoospermia occurs following a vasectomy (described later in this chapter). While most men are confident at the time of vasectomy that they will not desire any future fertility, approximately 5% change their mind. For these men, if semen has not been cryopreserved before vasectomy, two options exist to father more children who are biologically related to them – microsurgical reconstruction and surgical sperm retrieval in conjunction with IVF/ICSI. Which option to pursue depends on a number of factors about which couples must be carefully and dutifully informed. Because fertility-related procedures typically are not covered by most health insurance plans, it is important to try to help couples figure out what is the most cost-effective way to address the man's obstructive azoospermia. Should the couple proceed directly to sperm retrieval and IVF/ICSI, or should they proceed with microsurgical vasectomy reversal? **Factors in this decision can include the time since vasectomy, presence or absence of any female fertility factors (ovulatory status, tubal status, age of the woman, etc.), the desire for single or multiple children, and costs associated with each procedure** [17]. Vasectomy reversal is a more involved procedure for the man, while IVF/ICSI is more involved for the woman. **Generally, microsurgical reconstruction is more cost-effective when feasible (i.e., in the absence of a significant female factor or advanced maternal age)** [18].

A less common cause of iatrogenic vasal occlusion is a history of inguinal hernia repair. Particularly when mesh is used, inguinal hernia repair may result in a significant desmoplastic reaction around the inguinal ring that can cause obstruction of the vas deferens [19]. **It is important to bear this in mind if a young man of reproductive age with a symptomatic hernia desires repair, as he should be counseled about potential risks of fertility impairment.** If bilateral vasal occlusion results from bilateral inguinal hernia repairs, microsurgical reconstruction rarely is possible and surgical sperm retrieval with IVF/ICSI generally is recommended.

Regardless of the duration since a man's vasectomy, sperm production by the testis remains relatively normal, assuming no threat to his testicular function in the interim (e.g., chemotherapy). Techniques employed for microsurgical vasectomy reversal include vasovasostomy and epididymovasostomy. **The decision to perform either a vasovasostomy or epididymovasostomy generally can only be made at the time of reconstruction and depends on the presence of sperm in the testicular vas deferens as well as quality of vasal fluid.** There have been a number of predictors of success of vasectomy reversal, including time post-vasectomy [20], presence or absence of sperm granuloma, and length of the testicular end of the vas deferens [21]. It has been shown that when the testicular vasal remnant is greater than 2.7 cm that sperm will be found 94% of the time; however, when the testicular vasal remnant is less than 2.7 cm, sperm has been found only 15% of the time.

It has been repeatedly shown that use of the operating microscope affords the best outcomes when performing vasectomy reversal whether it be vasovasostomy or epididymovasostomy [20, 22]. The surgical set-up is vital to the success of the procedure, and having a well-coordinated operating team is essential for efficient and quality delivery of care (see Figure 3.4).

When sperm are seen in the testicular end of the vas deferens and vasovasostomy is planned, a two-layer microsurgical anastomosis of the vas deferens may offer superior outcomes (see Figure 3.5). The operating microscope is necessary when using nylon sutures as fine as 10-0 on the inner mucosal layer and 9-0 on the outer seromuscular layer. The diameter of a 10-0 nylon suture is approximately three to four times that of a red blood cell! **When bilateral microsurgical vasovasostomy can be performed, over 90% of patients will have sperm returning to the ejaculate** [22]. However, more importantly, the decision to perform a vasovasostomy or epididymovasostomy is most critical. Generally, vasovasostomy can be performed when whole motile or non-motile sperm are seen. If clear fluid is in the testicular vas deferens but no sperm, and if the interval has been less than 5 years, vasovasostomy generally is successful. When sperm heads and tails are found and the interval is less than 10 years, then microsurgical vasovasostomy is generally successful. **However, if there are no sperm seen and the quality of vasal fluid is thick, creamy, and pasty, then epididymovasostomy is necessary for a chance at successful vasectomy reversal.** When sperm heads are seen and vasal fluid is thick, it is unknown if vasovasostomy or epididymovasostomy affords the best outcomes.

(a)

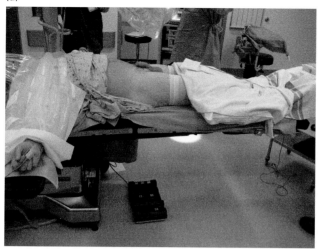

(b)

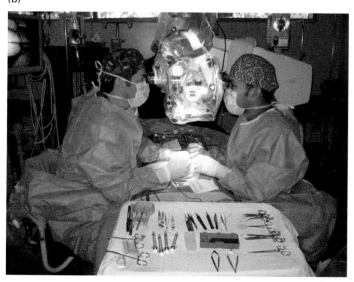

Figure 3.4 Setup for microsurgical vasectomy reversal. (a) The patient is positioned on the operating table so that the microsurgeon and assistant are able to sit with their legs under the table. (b) The microsurgeon and assistant sit across from each other on padded armchairs. The armchairs are draped with sterile surgical gowns. Microsurgical instruments and sutures are placed on a stand above the patient's thighs.

When epididymal obstruction has been identified at the time of vasectomy reversal then vasovasostomy is doomed for failure. In such cases, epididymovasostomy is the appropriate procedure to perform. The microsurgeon's training

(a)

(b)

(c)

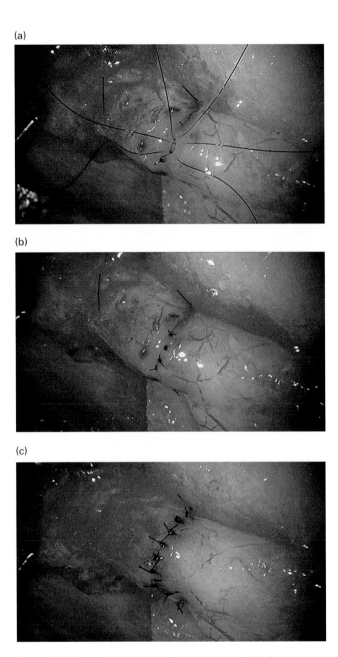

Figure 3.5 Microsurgical, two-layer vasovasostomy. (a) The posterior outer seromuscular and inner mucosal layers have been tied. The inner mucosal layer sutures of 10-0 nylon are individually placed anteriorly giving a "spider's web" appearance. (b) Inner mucosal sutures tied. (c) Outer seromuscular sutures of 9-0 nylon tied to create a watertight closure (see color plate section).

and level of comfort dictate the technique employed for epididymovasostomy whether it is end-to-end, end-to-side, or intussuscepted (see Figure 3.6). **The site for epididymal anastomosis should be carefully chosen, starting from the tail of the epididymis and moving towards the head as needed.** The closer to the tail and convoluted vas deferens, the larger the lumen of the epididymal tubules and the easier the anastomosis typically is. It is still debated whether sperm need to be seen in order for a successful epididymovasostomy to take place. Ideally, motile sperm are seen at the anastamotic site; however, whole non-motile sperm generally will suffice. If only sperm parts are identified, it is best to move to a more proximal tubule and check again for sperm quality. **In the event that a man needs to have a bilateral microsurgical epididymovasostomy, up to 70–80% of patients will have sperm return to their ejaculate** [23].

It must be emphasized that while there may be factors that can help predict the presence or absence of sperm in the testicular vas deferens prior to surgery, it is virtually unknown until vasal fluid is examined under light microscopy intraoperatively whether or not an epididymovasostomy will be necessary. **As such, the surgeon performing a microsurgical vasectomy reversal should have the training and skill to perform an epididymovasostomy when indicated.** This is particularly true if and when such a procedure is not covered by the patient's health insurance plan. **It is the duty and obligation of surgeons performing vasectomy reversals to disclose this information to their patients during preoperative counseling sessions.** Please see [3] (pp. 394–403) for more information about microsurgical vasectomy reversal techniques and outcomes.

Spermatogenic dysfunction

NOA refers to a problem with sperm production. Semen parameters typically include normal semen volume that is fructose positive with normal pH and no sperm in the ejaculate. There are a number of etiologies for NOA that can include a history of testicular torsion, testicular trauma, testicular cancer, varicocele, and cryptorchidism. It is important to bear in mind that sperm are found in roughly 20% of men with NOA (either motile or non-motile) in a centrifuged pellet sample [24]. This may be referred to as "cryptozoospermia" or "virtual azoospermia." Other causes of NOA can include genetic ones, such as Klinefelter syndrome, balanced chromosome translocations, and Y-chromosome microdeletions. **For this reason, part of the diagnostic algorithm for NOA includes checking both a karyotype and a Y-chromosome microdeletion test** (see [3], pp. 251–6 for more information about the genetics of NOA).

It has been found that approximately 15% of men with NOA and 10% of men with severe oligospermia (<5 million/ml) carry a Y-chromosome microdeletion. Less than 1% of men with sperm concentrations greater than 5 million/ml have Y-chromosome microdeletions [25]. A number of regions have been identified on the Y chromosome and have been termed azoospermic factor

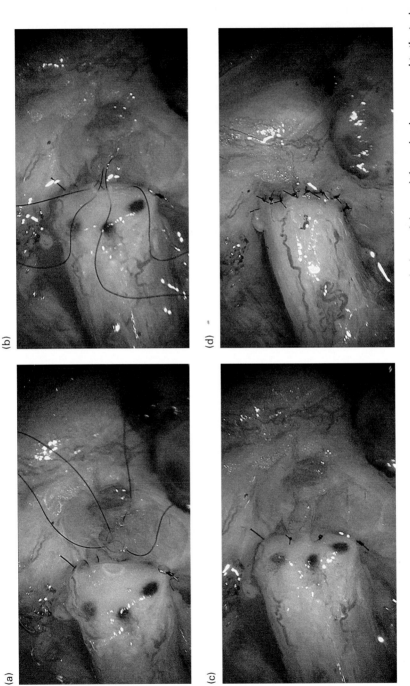

Figure 3.6 Microsurgical, intussusception epididymovasostomy. (a) The outer seromuscular layer of the vas deferens has been secured to the tunica of the epididymis with 9-0 nylon sutures. Double-armed 10-0 nylon sutures have been placed in an epididymal tubule. The tubule has been opened, and the presence of sperm has been confirmed. (b) The 10-0 nylon sutures are placed in the lumen of the vas deferens. (c) 10-0 nylon sutures tied, thereby intussuscepting the opened epididymal tubule into the lumen of the vas deferens. (d) The outer seromuscular layer of the vas deferens is anastamosed to the epididymal tunica with interrupted 9-0 nylon sutures (see color plate section).

(AZF) regions. While a number of regions have been identified, those of most clinical significance currently include AZF a, b, and c.

Finding the Y-chromosome microdeletion is important for a number of different reasons. First, it is always of interest to the patient and provider to have an explanation for why his sperm production is either absent or extremely low. **Additionally, if a Y-chromosome microdeletion is identified it can help predict the success in finding sperm on a testicular biopsy.** For example, sperm is detected in approximately 50% of men with the AZFc deletion at the time of testicular biopsy. Conversely, there are no reports of sperm in men with AZFb deletions, at testicular biopsy. Being a carrier of an AZFb deletion may obviate the need for a patient to undergo a potentially unnecessary testicular procedure [26].

There are a number of approaches for testicular sperm extraction (TESE). One approach is an open technique that can be performed either in the operating room under general anesthesia or conscious sedation, or in the office with a spermatic cord block. The procedure involves making a small opening on the scrotal skin and carrying this dissection through the tunica vaginalis and exposing the tunica albuginea. The tunica albuginea is then opened, seminiferous tubules are extruded and teased on to a slide using jeweler's forceps, and then the tissue is examined under a bench microscope. The opening(s) in the tunica albuginea are closed with running and locked sutures made of either absorbable or non-absorbable materials, and scrotal contents are closed in layers at the surgeon's preference using absorbable suture (see [3], color plates of figures 22.9, 22.10, and 22.11). **Another approach is microsurgical-TESE, which, using the operating microscope, allows for better visualization of areas within the testicle where spermatogenesis is likely to be present and thus minimizes the amount of tissue ultimately removed** [27] (see Figure 3.7).

When sperm are found in testis tissues in the setting of NOA, they can only be used in conjunction with advanced reproductive technologies, specifically IVF/ ICSI. A number of studies have demonstrated that clinical pregnancies can occur with sperm obtained from TESE in NOA [28]. Sperm obtained from TESE in the setting of NOA may be frozen if the embryology laboratory is familiar with cryopreserving testicular sperm. It is important for the urologist to be in close communication with the IVF laboratory to determine preferences in working with fresh versus frozen sperm in patients with NOA. Frozen sperm in the setting of obstructive azoospermia fair quite well when compared with fresh sperm. Please see [3] (pp. 412–15) for a detailed discussion of surgical sperm retrieval techniques for NOA.

Anejaculation

Any serious medical illness or surgery can result in impaired testicular function and disruption of normal ejaculatory function. Such conditions can include high fevers or debilitating illnesses, retroperitoneal surgery, pelvic injury, previous history of a bladder outlet obstruction procedure such as Y-V plasty, or TURP. When a man undergoes a retroperitoneal lymph node

(a)

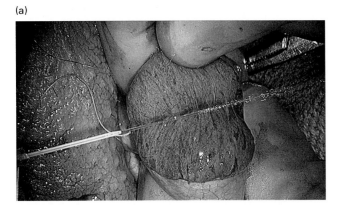

(b)

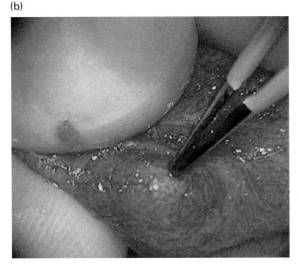

Figure 3.7 Microdissection testicular sperm extraction (micro-TESE). (a) The tunica albuginea is opened along the equator of the testicle under low power. (b) Under higher-power optical magnification, seminiferous tubules that are believed to have active spermatogenesis (at tips of bipolar forceps) are seen as being "full" relative to the smaller "empty" tubules around them (see color plate section).

dissection in the setting of a non-seminomatous germ cell tumor, such a procedure can potentially damage the thoracic and lumbar sympathetic chains and pelvic plexus that control ejaculatory function. Although advances in nerve-sparing templates for retroperitoneal lymph node dissections have resulted in an increased number of men who maintain their ejaculatory function postoperatively, this surgery nevertheless can be a risk factor for ejaculatory failure. **Sperm cryopreservation before cancer therapy is considered standard of care and must be discussed and offered to men preoperatively before undergoing such procedures or treatments that threaten a man's future fertility potential** [29].

If ejaculatory failure occurs following retroperitoneal lymph node dissection or other low-abdominal or retroperitoneal surgery, certain medical approaches may be offered, although success generally is marginal. Sympathomimetic agents such as pseudoephedrine and imipramine may improve ejaculatory function, as these medications can increase smooth muscle tone of the bladder neck. Penile vibratory stimulation may also be attempted (see [3], pp. 460–1, figures 26.2, 26.3, and 26.4). Penile vibratory stimulation requires an intact spinal loop, and therefore works best in men with spinal cord injuries where the level of injury is T10 or above [30]. In some patients, semen may be expressed by aggressive massaging of the seminal vesicles. **However, if antegrade ejaculation is not possible with medical therapy or with penile vibratory stimulation, then the best treatment of ejaculatory failure in this setting is transrectal EEJ** [31].

EEJ is performed with men either in the lateral decubitus or dorsal lithotomy position (see [3], p. 463, figure 26.7). Preoperative antibiotics and urinary alkalinizing agents are given. The bladder is emptied with a catheter and then washed with a sperm wash media or human tubal fluid provided by the reproductive endocrinology clinic and andrology laboratory performing the subsequent treatment for the couple, either IUI or IVF/ICSI. About 30 ml of sperm wash media are left in the bladder. The EEJ probe is placed in the rectum to obtain an interface anteriorly with the accessory sex organs. The electrode power is gradually increased in a pulsatile manner until a rhythmic pelvic floor contraction is elicited. Any antegrade semen is collected. If none is present, then the bladder is catheterized and the previously placed sperm wash media is collected for analysis. **Following this procedure, it is important to perform a rectoscopy to evaluate any burn injuries to the rectal mucosa.**

When men are sensate, EEJ requires a general anesthetic. For men who are completely insensate (i.e., following a complete spinal cord injury), this procedure may be performed in an office setting. Depending on the level of spinal cord injury, the patient may or may not be at risk for reflex autonomic dysfunction and may need to be carefully monitored for blood pressure and pulse abnormalities. **Premedication with vasoactive agents such as sublingual nifedipine can help prevent such autonomic dysreflexia, particularly when the level of injury is T6 or above.**

While transrectal EEJ is almost always successful, semen quality is almost always impaired. When IUI is possible based on semen parameters, the success rates are generally lower than for other couples undergoing IUI. However, success rates with IVF/ICSI are generally equivalent to other couples [32].

Another application of EEJ can be in men or boys before undergoing either chemotherapy or radiotherapy that can be damaging to their spermatogenic function. If these patients are incapable of producing semen samples for sperm cryopreservation, then this technique can be employed. General anesthesia is necessary in such cases.

The cost-effectiveness of EEJ for men with ejaculatory failure generally depends on whether or not a general anesthetic is required. For sensate individuals who need general anesthesia, EEJ may be cost-prohibitive, particularly if used in conjunction with IUIs, as they generally require a number of cycles before achieving pregnancy. For insensate patients in whom adequate numbers of total motile sperm may be obtained via EEJ in the office, this approach in conjunction with IUI may ultimately be more cost-effective than surgical sperm retrieval with IVF/ICSI [33]. Ultimately, the couple must decide what path they wish to pursue, and this often depends on differences in regional costs and availability of assisted reproductive technologies. Please see [3] (pp. 454–69) for more detailed discussions of ejaculatory dysfunction and treatment.

Vasectomy

Approximately 500,000 vasectomies are performed every year in the United States. **It is the most common and most effective surgical means of male contraception.** Vasectomy is considered nearly 100% effective, and a paternity rate with postoperative azoospermia is reported to be 1 in 2000.

Vasectomy is usually performed in the office using a local anesthetic but may be performed in the operating room under a formal anesthetic upon request or if it is difficult to feel the vas deferens in the clinic. Vasectomy is performed through a small opening in the scrotal skin. **Most urologists use the "no-scalpel" technique using instruments specifically designed for manipulating the vas deferens.** The skin and vas deferens are first anesthetized with a local anesthetic, and the vas deferens is identified and tied or clipped usually in two locations. A small segment of the vas deferens is removed. The small opening in the scrotum is then closed and the identical procedure is performed on the other side. **Histologic confirmation generally is not required, as the pathological findings do not obviate the need to check postoperative semen samples.**

A number of techniques of vasal occlusion exist, including suture ligature, hemoclips, intraluminal needle electrocautery, and fascial interposition. However, no technique is 100% effective [34]. **Additionally, no standard exists by which a patient may be declared sterile.** Checking at least one, if not two semen analyses, separated by about a month, beginning about 2–3 months post-vasectomy is recommended [35]. Couples need to continue using their current method(s) of birth control until these samples are obtained and azoospermia is documented.

Patients and providers need to be aware of a number of key points about vasectomies. Generally, they are low-risk procedures. Rare but potential problems include hematoma, infection, testicular pain, testicular injury, formation of sperm granuloma, failure for sperm to clear from the ejaculate, and recanalization of the vas deferens. Vasectomy is safe and does not interfere with a man's sexual drive, virility, or his ability to have or enjoy sex. The amount of ejaculate is virtually unchanged after a vasectomy as the sperm from the testicles make up only about 5% of the total volume. The rest of the seminal fluid is made distal to the vasectomy site in the prostate gland and seminal vesicles. Vasectomy does not protect men from sexually transmitted disease. **Finally, the most critical aspect** of vasectomy is careful and thorough patient counseling with emphasis on compliance with obtaining postoperative semen analyses, as studies suggest that only 70–80% of men actually have their semen checked after their vasectomy.

Please see [3] (pp. 474–80) for a more detailed discussion of vasectomy.

REFERENCES

[1] Pryor JL, Howards SS. Varicocele. *Urol Clin North Am* 1987; **14**(3): 499–513.

[2] Fretz PC, Sandlow JI. Varicocele: current concepts in pathophysiology, diagnosis, and treatment. *Urol Clin North Am* 2002; **29**(4): 921–37.

[3] Lipshultz L, Howards S, Niederberger C, eds. *Infertility in the Male*, 4th edn (Cambridge, Cambridge University Press, 2009).

[4] Dubin L, Amelar RD. Varicocele size and results of varicocelectomy in selected subfertile men with varicocele. *Fertil Steril* 1970; **21**(8): 606–9.

[5] Chiou RK, Anderson JC, Wobig RK, *et al.* Color Doppler ultrasound criteria to diagnose varicoceles: correlation of a new scoring system with physical examination. *Urology* 1997; **50**(6): 953–6.

[6] Goldstein M, Eid JF. Elevation of intratesticular and scrotal skin surface temperature in men with varicocele. *J Urol* 1989; **142**(3): 743–5.

[7] Agger P, Johnsen SG. Quantitative evaluation of testicular biopsies in varicocele. *Fertil Steril* 1978; **29**: 52–7.

[8] Goldstein M, Gilbert BR, Dicker AP, Dwosh J, Gnecco C. Microsurgical inguinal varicocelectomy with delivery of the testis: an artery and lymphatic sparing technique. *J Urol* 1992; **148**(6): 1808–11.

[9] Daitch JA, Bedaiwy MA, Pasqualotto EB, *et al.* Varicocelectomy improves intrauterine insemination success rates in men with varicocele. *J Urol* 2001; **165**(5): 1510–13.

[10] The influence of varicocele on parameters of fertility in a large group of men presenting to infertility clinics. World Health Organization. *Fertil Steril* 1992; **57**(6): 1289–93.

[11] Halden W, White RI, Jr. Outpatient embolotherapy of varicocele. *Urol Clin North Am* 1987; **14**: 137–44.

[12] Morag B, Rubinstein ZJ, Goldwasser B, Yerushalmi A, Lunnenfeld B. Percutaneous venography and occlusion in the management of spermatic varicoceles. *AJR Am J Roentgenol* 1984; **143**(3): 635–40.

[13] Jarow JP. Transrectal ultrasonography in the diagnosis and management of ejaculatory duct obstruction. *J Androl* 1996; **17**(5): 467–72.

[14] Jarow JP. Seminal vesicle aspiration in the management of patients with ejaculatory duct obstruction. *J Urol* 1994; **152**(3): 899–901.

[15] Purohit RS, Wu DS, Shinohara K, Turek PJ. A prospective comparison of 3 diagnostic methods to evaluate ejaculatory duct obstruction. *J Urol* 2004; **171**: 232–5; discussion 5–6.

[16] Meacham RB, Hellerstein DK, Lipshultz LI. Evaluation and treatment of ejaculatory duct obstruction in the infertile male. *Fertil Steril* 1993; **59**(2): 393–7.

[17] Fuchs EF, Burt RA. Vasectomy reversal performed 15 years or more after vasectomy: correlation of pregnancy outcome with partner age and with pregnancy

results of in vitro fertilization with intracytoplasmic sperm injection. *Fertil Steril* 2002; **77**(3): 516–19.

[18] Meng MV, Greene KL, Turek PJ. Surgery or assisted reproduction? A decision analysis of treatment costs in male infertility. *J Urol* 2005; **174**(5): 1926–31; discussion 31.

[19] Shin D, Lipshultz LI, Goldstein M, *et al.* Herniorrhaphy with polypropylene mesh causing inguinal vasal obstruction: a preventable cause of obstructive azoospermia. *Ann Surg* 2005; **241**(4): 553–8.

[20] Belker AM, Thomas AJ, Jr., Fuchs EF, Konnak JW, Sharlip ID. Results of 1,469 microsurgical vasectomy reversals by the Vasovasostomy Study Group. *J Urol* 1991; **145**(3): 505–11.

[21] Witt MA, Heron S, Lipshultz LI. The post-vasectomy length of the testicular vasal remnant: a predictor of surgical outcome in microscopic vasectomy reversal. *J Urol* 1994; **151**(4): 892–4.

[22] Lee L, McLoughlin MG. Vasovasostomy: a comparison of macroscopic and microscopic techniques at one institution. *Fertil Steril* 1980; **33**: 54–5.

[23] Schiff J, Chan P, Li PS, Finkelberg S, Goldstein M. Outcome and late failures compared in 4 techniques of microsurgical vasoepididymostomy in 153 consecutive men. *J Urol* 2005; **174**(2): 651–5; quiz 801.

[24] Jaffe TM, Kim ED, Hoekstra TH, Lipshultz LI. Sperm pellet analysis: a technique to detect the presence of sperm in men considered to have azoospermia by routine semen analysis. *J Urol* 1998; **159**(5): 1548–50.

[25] Pryor JL, Kent-First M, Muallem A, *et al.* Microdeletions in the Y chromosome of infertile men. *N Engl J Med* 1997; **336**(8): 534–9.

[26] Krausz C, Forti G, McElreavey K. The Y chromosome and male fertility and infertility. *Int J Androl* 2003; **26**(2): 70–5.

[27] Okada H, Dobashi M, Yamazaki T, *et al.* Conventional versus microdissection testicular sperm extraction for nonobstructive azoospermia. *J Urol* 2002; **168**(3): 1063–7.

[28] Schlegel PN. Testicular sperm extraction: microdissection improves sperm yield with minimal tissue excision. *Hum Reprod* 1999; **14**: 131–5.

[29] Lee SJ, Schover LR, Partridge AH, *et al.* American Society of Clinical Oncology recommendations on fertility preservation in cancer patients. *J Clin Oncol* 2006; **24**(18): 2917–31.

[30] Kafetsoulis A, Brackett NL, Ibrahim E, Attia GR, Lynne CM. Current trends in the treatment of infertility in men with spinal cord injury. *Fertil Steril* 2006; **86**(4): 781–9.

[31] Seager SW, Halstead LS. Fertility options and success after spinal cord injury. *Urol Clin North Am* 1993; **20**(3): 543–8.

[32] Brackett NL, Abae M, Padron OF, Lynne CM. Treatment by assisted conception of severe male factor infertility due to spinal cord injury or other neurologic impairment. *J Assist Reprod Genet* 1995; **12**(3): 210–16.

[33] Ohl DA, Wolf LJ, Menge AC, *et al.* Electroejaculation and assisted reproductive technologies in the treatment of anejaculatory infertility. *Fertil Steril* 2001; **76**(6): 1249–55.

[34] Maatman TJ, Aldrin L, Carothers GG. Patient noncompliance after vasectomy. *Fertil Steril* 1997; **68**(3): 552–5.

[35] Barone MA, Nazerali H, Cortes M, *et al.* A prospective study of time and number of ejaculations to azoospermia after vasectomy by ligation and excision. *J Urol* 2003; **170**(3): 892–6.

4

Non-surgical therapy

Randall B. Meacham, MD

Introduction

Male infertility is a relatively common condition, and can be a source of tremendous anxiety and stress among those who suffer from it. Approximately 15% of couples will be unable to conceive following 1 year of unprotected intercourse. In 50% of such couples, a male factor will be responsible for their inability to conceive, either alone or in combination with a female fertility factor (see [1], p. 153). Most men found to be subfertile had no previous suspicion that they would encounter problems establishing a family. **The news that a man is unable to father a child is often a blow to his self-esteem and can foster feelings of desperation and despair.** In situations such as this, the patient and his partner understandably "want something done" about their inability to conceive and often feel stressed in their efforts to conceive.

The past several decades have led to a significantly better understanding of male reproductive physiology, thus providing improved tools for treating some causes of male infertility. Constant refinement in operative technique has led to better outcomes among men with fertility lesions that are amenable to surgical correction. Still, a significant number of men who present for the management of subfertility will not be found to have a correctable lesion. Such men, however, are often no less convinced that something must be done to improve their prospects for conception. The emotional energy of such patients, in combination with the understandable desire on the part of those involved in the care of fertility patients to offer hope, has led to the broad application of many poorly supported and potentially counterproductive efforts in the pharmacologic management of male infertility. If you treat enough male fertility patients, you will encounter a remarkable number of such quasi-therapeutic regimens that have been

An Introduction to Male Reproductive Medicine, ed. Craig Niederberger. Published by Cambridge University Press. © Cambridge University Press 2011.

prescribed by previous practitioners. **While many such therapeutic strategies are based on valid physiologic principles, few have well-designed, double-blind, placebo-controlled trial data to support their use. The medications involved are often expensive and they may divert a couple who would benefit from the application of assisted reproductive technologies from pursuing that approach while they embark on a protracted course of medical treatment.**

In the course of providing fertility care, you will have many opportunities to ask yourself, am I considering this treatment because I have good reason to believe that it will materially improve my patient's chances for conception, or am I considering it because I have "nothing else to offer." If your answer is the latter, you should carefully consider whether or not suggesting such therapy constitutes a service to your patient. In most cases, detailed discussion of the physiology of male infertility with emphasis on factors that are operative in an individual patient's clinical scenario will provide comfort to a previously confused and frightened individual. If no treatment is available, stating that fact in an honest and caring fashion will frequently be received with equanimity and gratitude on the part of the patient and their partner. Further, if you can offer no specific therapy that will enhance your patient's fertility potential, a factual discussion will offer him the chance to move on to other opportunities such as the application of androgen replacement therapy (if the clinical scenario permits), the use of donor sperm, or adoption.

Having said all of this, there are certainly situations where the application of non-surgical therapy will significantly enhance the potential for a subfertile man to father a child. In this chapter, I will discuss a number of specific therapeutic modalities aimed at the management of defined causes of male infertility.

Medications and substances to avoid among men seeking to establish a pregnancy

Men who are concerned about fertility often worry extensively about environmental factors that may diminish it. They (or their partners) may establish an overly strict regimen that prohibits activities likely to have little impact on fertility. **Such men may be avoiding physical exercise, exposure to warm showers, modest levels of caffeine, use of laptop computers, etc., based on the impression that such factors may harm their chances of conception. This alteration in daily activity may in itself add significant stress to an already difficult situation while offering little or no reproductive benefit.**

Certain medications, however, should be avoided during attempts at conception. Prominent among these is supplemental testosterone. Androgen replacement therapy is gaining significant attention as a possible treatment for ailments ranging from lack of libido to increased body fat to depression and decreased mental acuity. Given the broad application of this therapeutic modality, it is not uncommon to find that patients being treated for male fertility concerns are using androgen replacement therapy. Moreover, men dealing with fertility concerns may be placed on androgen replacement therapy by well-meaning practitioners in an effort to promote testicular function. Given the fact that exogenous testosterone suppresses luteinizing hormone (LH) production by the pituitary, the use of supplemental testosterone dramatically decreases endogenous testosterone production and, therefore, intratesticular levels of testosterone (see [1], pp. 446–7). This decrease in intra-testicular androgen levels suppresses spermatogenesis, thereby dramatically decreasing sperm production. Male fertility patients who are using androgen supplementation should be encouraged to discontinue this therapy. It will likely take several months before they regain their previous levels of spermatogenesis, but such patients will often realize a "miraculous" recovery of their fertility status once this has been accomplished.

Some men who using androgen replacement therapy will become excessively symptomatic when they discontinue treatment, or their baseline serum testosterone may be sufficiently low as to raise concern that decreased androgen production is exerting a negative impact on their fertility. In such cases, use of clomiphene citrate will often allow restoration of testosterone levels to the normal or near-normal range (see [1], pp. 438–53). Clomiphene therapy can generally be initiated at a dose of 50 mg/day or every other day. The dose can then be titrated to achieve a serum testosterone level within the normal range. It should be noted that in some cases of severe testicular failure, the testes might not produce sufficient testosterone in response to clomiphene administration to achieve the desired effect. In this case, elevated LH can guide whether clomiphene is likely to be successful, with levels above 25 IU/l indicating a low chance of success.

Other medications that may have a negative impact on male fertility include cimetidine, antihypertensive medications, calcium channel blockers, spironolactone, and angiotensin-converting enzyme inhibitors (see [1], p. 430).

Men attempting to father a child should also be advised to minimize the use of alcohol, tobacco, marijuana, and other recreational drugs (see [1], pp. 430–1). While there are limited data available to define what level of exposure to such agents will have a negative impact on male fertility, it makes sense for men who have marginal semen quality to avoid these substances to the extent possible. In general, I suggest to my patients that "what is bad for them, is likely to be bad for their sperm."

Infections

Management of genitourinary infections may play a role in the managing of male fertility patients. *Chlamydia trachomatis* is a remarkably common pathogen identified as a possible causative factor in male infertility (see [1], p. 431). The pathogenic role of chlamydia infection in male infertility is not entirely clear. Chlamydia infection may directly impact sperm function, induce increased numbers of leukocytes in the semen, or contribute to ductal obstruction. Suspicion of chlamydial infection may arise when more than 1 million leukocytes/ml of semen are noted during male fertility evaluation. In such cases, further evaluation for chlamydia may be appropriate, although empiric antimicrobial therapy might be a more practical approach. Genitourinary infections and their treatments are discussed in Chapter 5 of this book.

Management of hypogonadotropic hypogonadism

Kallmann's syndrome, while rare, is an excellent example of a male fertility lesion that is often amenable to non-surgical therapy. This syndrome is associated with defects such as anosmia or hyposmia and is most commonly inherited in an X-linked pattern (see [1], p. 433). As with other forms of hypogonadotropic hypogonadism, the management of Kallmann's syndrome hinges on therapeutic replacement of gonadotropins, allowing adequate production of testosterone and initiation of spermatogenesis. Therapy is typically initiated using the LH analog human chorionic gonadotropin (hCG) at a dose of 2000 units subcutaneously three times per week to 5000 units twice weekly. The dose of hCG is titrated to achieve a serum testosterone level within an acceptable range. hCG administration is continued for 6 months at which time semen analysis is obtained. If sperm are not present, follicle-stimulating hormone therapy is begun using human menopausal gonadotropin at a dose of 75 units subcutaneously three times per week. An alternative approach to the management of this condition is the use of a GnRH infusion pump. This approach is more technologically demanding and is typically used among men who do not respond to therapy using hCG and human menopausal gonadotropin (see [1], pp. 432–3).

Androgen replacement therapy

While exogenous testosterone causes a precipitous fall in the production of testosterone in the testes, other strategies may be used to increase testicular synthesis of testosterone should total or bioavailable testosterone be found to be low (see Chapter 2 of this book). As the endocrine moiety primarily exerting negative feedback on pituitary LH secretion is estradiol, inhibitors of estradiol such as clomiphene and tamoxifen will increase both serum and intratesticular testosterone levels.

Another strategy that might increase intratesticular and serum testosterone is to administer inhibitors of aromatase, the enzyme that converts testosterone to estradiol. This is particularly useful when elevated estradiol accompany depressed testosterone levels. Raman and Schlegel proposed a ratio of testosterone (in ng/dl) to estradiol (in pg/ml) of 10:1 to suggest use of aromatase inhibitors, such as anastrozole or testolactone [2].

Hyperprolactinemia

Hyperprolactinemia is another cause of male infertility that is often amenable to non-surgical therapy. Elevated levels of prolactin may impair male fertility based on multiple pathways. Prolactin inhibits the action of LH on Leydig cells and prolactin receptors are found in the first layer of the seminiferous epithelium – suggesting that prolactin may have a direct effect on sperm production [3]. Prolactin-secreting adenomas are the most common functional pituitary tumors (4). Ninety percent of adenomas are microadenomas (less than 10 mm in size) with the remaining 10% being macroadenomas (greater than 10 mm in size). Symptomatic prolactinomas are more common among women than men. This may be because symptoms that occur in women are more easily identified than those seen in men [4]. Men suffering from prolactin-secreting adenomas may report symptoms, including headaches, visual abnormalities, galactorrhea, erectile dysfunction, and decreased libido (see [1], p. 433). Male patients with increased prolactin levels will frequently demonstrate abnormally low serum testosterone levels. Bringing prolactin levels into the normal range will often reverse such hypogonadism. Male infertility patients presenting with hyperprolactinemia should be evaluated via pituitary MRI to determine the presence and size of the tumor if one is present. In general, the presence of a macroadenoma is associated with serum prolactin levels greater than 200 µg/l (see [1], p. 433). **Management of hyperprolactinemia is usually based upon the presence and size of an adenoma.** Patients who have a normal MRI and those with microadenomas can be treated with dopaminergic agonists, including bromocriptine and cabergoline. **Cabergoline has been shown to be superior to bromocriptine in the treatment of hyperprolactinemia because it is more effective in lowering prolactin levels and reducing tumor size, while causing fewer side-effects. Moreover, patients treated with cabergoline are more likely to achieve permanent remission and successful withdrawal of medication than those treated with bromocriptine** [5]. Patients with macroadenomas should be referred to a neurosurgeon for consideration of tumor ablation. Recent experience has indicated that an endoscopic approach to such ablation procedures is both effective and well tolerated.

Effective management of hyperprolactinemia can result in improvement in symptoms associated with this condition and in semen quality. The diagnosis of hyperprolactinemia should, therefore, be kept in mind when evaluating subfertile men who demonstrate decreased androgen levels or symptoms associated with a pituitary mass.

Use of clomiphene citrate before testis biopsy

A particularly interesting application of pharmacotherapy in the management of male infertility is the use of clomiphene citrate before testis biopsy in the management of azoospermic men suffering from primary testicular failure. The rationale behind such therapy is based on the mechanism of action of clomiphene, which induces increased gonadotropin release by the pituitary, thereby increasing testosterone production by the testis, and possibly enhancing spermatogenesis. While clomiphene citrate has long been employed empirically in an effort to increase sperm production in subfertile men, its empirical application has generally not been supported by robust clinical data. A recent study, however, evaluated the use of clomiphene before performing testis biopsy among men diagnosed with non-obstructive testicular failure. Forty-two men with this condition were treated with clomiphene citrate, titrating the dose to achieve serum testosterone levels of 600–800 ng/dl. **After 3–9 months of treatment, 64.3% demonstrated sperm in the ejaculate. All patients who underwent testis biopsy were found to have sufficient sperm to undergo ICSI.** Should these results be confirmed in larger, controlled studies, such treatment would potentially obviate the need for testis biopsy in a number of patients and possibly improve the outcomes for patients who undergo this procedure [6].

Choice of undergarments

A topic worth discussing based on the sheer frequency with which it is brought up by patients is the type of undergarment that male fertility patients should be advised to wear. For many years, it has been held as a matter of faith by many members of the general public that boxer shorts allow the testes to maintain a lower temperature and therefore are beneficial to male fertility when compared with snug-fitting briefs. Some medical practitioners also recommend that men interested in fertility switch from briefs to boxers. A characteristic scene frequently arises in the office of the male fertility specialist. A very uncomfortable looking man arrives for evaluation. Already stricken with embarrassment over the need to discuss the details of his reproductive life, he must then disrobe for the physical examination. One can only sympathize as the patient lowers his pants to reveal a pair of huge, ill fitting, garishly decorated boxer shorts recently purchased by his well-meaning partner. Such garments (which often seem to display the name of a professional sports team or depictions of some species of animal – or both) only serve to add additional stress to an already stressful period in the man's life. While the wearing of loose-fitting undershorts may make some degree of physiological sense, their use has never been supported in any rigorous scientific fashion. One illuminating study compared the use of boxer shorts versus briefs in a crossover study that compared scrotal skin temperature and semen parameters among men wearing the two types of underwear. **No difference was noted among the two groups, indicating that the choice of underwear is purely a matter of aesthetics and comfort rather than reproductive function** (7).

Empiric non-surgical therapy for male infertility

A seemingly endless array of empiric therapies have been directed at the improvement of male reproductive capacity. Substances, including antiestrogen agents, aromatase inhibitors, gonadotropins, L-carnitine, antioxidants, and a variety of other compounds have been employed for years with little conclusive evidence that they consistently improve either semen quality or pregnancy rates. A comprehensive review of empiric non-surgical therapy for male infertility can be found in [1] (chapter 25). The use of complementary and alternative treatment modalities is also quite prevalent among couples seeking to establish a pregnancy [8]. While it is difficult to say conclusively whether complementary treatments can have a positive impact on fertility, once again, little high-quality data exist to support this approach.

REFERENCES

[1] Lipshultz L, Howards S, Niederberger C, eds. *Infertility in the Male*, 4th edn (Cambridge, Cambridge University Press, 2009).
[2] Raman JD, Schlegel PN. Aromatase inhibitors for male infertility. *J Urol* 2002; **167**: 624–9.
[3] Nishimura K, Matsumiya K, Tsuboniwa N, *et al.* Bromocriptine for infertile males with mild hyperprolactinemia: hormonal and spermatogenic effects. *Arch Androl* 1999; **43**: 207–13.
[4] Schlechte JA. Long-term management of prolactinomas. *J Clin Endocrinol Metab* 2007; **92**(8): 2861–5.
[5] Gillam MP, Molich ME, Lombardi G, *et al.* Advances in the treatment of prolactinomas. *Endocr Rev* 2006; **27**(5): 485–534.
[6] Hussein A, Ozgok Y, Ross L, Niederberger C. Clomiphene administration for cases of nonobstructive azoospermia: a multicenter study. *J Androl* 2005; **26**: 787–91.
[7] Munkelwitz R, Gilbert BR. Are boxer shorts really better? A critical analysis of the role of underwear type in male subfertility. *J Urol* 1998; **160**(4): 1329–33.
[8] Smith JF, Eisenberg ML, Millstein SG, *et al.* The use of complementary and alternative fertility treatment in couples seeking fertility care: data from a prospective cohort in the United States. *Fertil Steril* 2010; **93**(7): 2169.

5

Male reproductive immunology

Robert E. Brannigan, MD

Introduction

Normal male reproductive potential relies upon the effective production of sperm in the testes and subsequent delivery of sperm into the female reproductive tract. As is detailed in other chapters of this text, a number of pathophysiological abnormalities can lead to disruption of sperm production or function and result in male infertility. Among these conditions is a subset involving infection, inflammation, and immune-mediated changes. In this chapter, we will discuss this group of conditions, including their causes, impact on male fertility, and available treatment options.

Infections of the male reproductive tract

The male reproductive tract is not a single anatomical entity. Rather, it is an amalgamation of several different physical structures, each with its own unique role in furthering the process of sperm production, maturation, and delivery to the female reproductive tract. **Despite the unique nature of each of the male reproductive tract components, they are all susceptible to infection and/or inflammation**. In each instance, the pathophysiological changes can lead to a significant decline in reproductive capability (see [1], pp. 295–7). Below we will detail specific sites of inflammation and infection within the male reproductive tract, characterizing each to provide a framework for arriving at the proper diagnosis, treatment, and counseling options for the affected patient.

An Introduction to Male Reproductive Medicine, ed. Craig Niederberger. Published by Cambridge University Press. © Cambridge University Press 2011.

Sites of male reproductive tract inflammation and infection

Urethra

The urethra is the portal to the genitourinary tract, and as such is the first line of anatomical defense against bacterial and viral pathogens. The female urethra is only 4 cm in length, and this short distance provides better opportunities for outside organisms to access the bladder and other urinary tract structures. This short distance is one key reason why women are more prone to urinary tract infections than men. In contrast, the urethra in men is typically 22 cm in length, and this length is a critical factor in preventing invading pathogens access to the rest of the genitourinary tract structures [2]. The urethra is further protected by the regular, periodic flow of urine, which helps to physically flush away organisms that may have made their way into the distal aspect of the urethra. **Despite the safeguards of length and urine flow, the male urethra is still at risk of developing infections. This condition, called urethritis, poses a number of threats to male reproduction.** The infecting organisms can migrate more proximally in the male, involving the epididymis (epididymitis) and the testes (orchitis), conditions that will be detailed later in this chapter. Anatomical changes can develop after urethritis, namely urethral stricture disease. Urethral strictures can predispose to additional, future urinary tract infections and, in severe cases, cause impaired delivery of sperm from the man during ejaculation. Finally, and of extreme importance, is the fact that urethritis can potentially be transmitted to the female sexual partner. **The resultant harmful effects of sexually transmitted infections to the female partner may include pelvic inflammatory disease, tubo-ovarian abscess, and obstruction of the fallopian tubes. In addition to the risk of significantly impairing her fertility potential, these conditions can also pose long-lasting, serious threats to the female partner's overall health.**

Urethritis typically arises from sexually transmitted organisms and is divided into two main types: gonococcal urethritis (due to infection by *Neisseria gonorrhoeae*) and non-gonococcal urethritis (due to infection by *Chlamydia trachomatis*, *Mycoplasma* species, and *Trichomonas vaginalis*). Co-infection with both *Neisseria gonorrhoeae* and *Chlamydia trachomatis* is a very real concern and occurs in about 30% of cases of urethritis. Upon presentation, patients with urethritis often complain of dysuria and urethral discharge. It is important to keep in mind though that infected individuals may be completely free of clinical symptoms. This is particularly important when considering the testing of sexual partners of infected individuals. **In other words, the testing of sexual partners of patients with urethritis is essential, because clinical signs and symptoms may be altogether absent despite an active, ongoing infection.**

The diagnosis of urethritis is typically made via:

1. Gram stain of urethral fluid (>4 white blood cell [WBC]/high-power field is positive).

2. WBC microscopic assessment of the first few milliliters of a voided urine sample (>15 WBC/high-power field is positive).
3. Endourethral culture, polymerase chain reaction, or enzyme-linked immunosorbent assay laboratory techniques (specific organism localization is positive) [3].

When a diagnosis of urethritis is entertained, clinicians should consider treating (empirically) for both gonococcal and non-gonococcal organisms, as concurrent infection with both categories are common. Typical therapy includes a single dose of ceftriaxone with a 7-day course of doxycycline or a 2-g dose of azithromycin.

Prostate

The prostate contributes a significant percentage of fluid to the male ejaculate. Infection and/or inflammation of this structure can have a markedly negative effect on semen quality. **"Prostatitis" is a very broad, heterogeneous term, referring to an array of conditions that are subcategorized using National Institutes of Health (NIH) Criteria.** We will briefly discuss each of these subgroups and their impact on reproduction below [4].

Acute bacterial prostatitis (*NIH Type I prostatitis*) is defined as prostate inflammation in the setting of an acute bacterial prostate infection, which is usually accompanied by a fever. The infecting organism is usually a uropathogen, and access to the prostate can arise via the urinary tract, pelvic lymphatics, or hematogenous spread. Diagnosis can be aided by culturing the urine (patients will often have concurrent cystitis) or seminal fluid. **While prostate fluid (expressed prostate secretions) obtained by prostate massage can also provide valuable clinical information, prostate massage should *not* be performed on patients with accompanying fevers or chills, as bacterial translocation into the bloodstream (bacteremia) and sepsis can result. This string of events can have potentially life-threatening effects on the patient.** Common symptoms of acute bacterial prostatitis include lower urinary tract symptoms (frequency, urgency, hesitancy, dysuria), pelvic or perineal pain, and generalized systemic symptoms (fatigue, myalgia, fever, and chills). Initially, broad-spectrum antibiotic therapy is generally indicated followed by a 2–3-week course of antimicrobial therapy tailored to culture data. This approach is usually effective in resolving uncomplicated cases. Anti-inflammatory therapy can be added to help resolve this condition as well. In acute prostatitis complicated by a prostatic abscess, transurethral drainage of the abscess is often needed to facilitate resolution of this disease process.

Chronic bacterial prostatitis (*NIH Type II prostatitis*) is heralded by the presence of prostate inflammation and bacterial infection that localizes to the prostate. Responsible organisms typically include the uropathogenic gram-negative organisms (*Escherichia coli*, *Klebsiella* species, *Proteus* species, *Pseudomonas* species) and gram-positive *Enterococcus* species. **Chronic bacterial prostatitis differs from acute bacterial prostatitis in that the former** is typically *not* accompanied by constitutional symptoms such as fever, chills, myalgia, and malaise. Lower urinary tract symptoms and pelvic or perineal pain are commonly present, though. An extended course of antibiotics (4–6 weeks) is often necessary, with agents such as fluoroquinolones or trimethoprim–sulfamethoxazole. **Patients on fluoroquinolone therapy should be followed closely though, as prolonged courses of treatment can result in tendinitis and tendon rupture.**

Chronic pelvic pain syndrome (NIH Type III prostatitis) is defined as patients having voiding symptoms and pelvic pain in the absence of detectable bacterial infection. NIH Type IIIA prostatitis (inflammatory type) is relevant for our discussion in the context of infertility, as these patients have increased WBC levels in prostate secretions obtained by prostate massage (expressed prostate secretions) or in the ejaculate. Later in this chapter, we will more specifically address the adverse effects of WBCs on semen quality and sperm function. Anti-inflammatory therapy is certainly a relevant treatment consideration for men with NIH Type IIIA prostatitis, or any form of prostatitis that results in increased WBC levels in semen. We should note that NIH Type IIIB prostatitis, noninflammatory type, is highly prevalent but is not particularly germane to this discussion regarding fertility. Patients with this condition have pelvic and perineal pain symptoms but do not have elevated levels of WBCs in the prostate fluid or semen. NIH Type IIIB prostatitis is believed by many to be due to pelvic muscular tension.

Asymptomatic inflammatory prostatitis (NIH Type IV prostatitis) is an incidental finding of prostate inflammation on prostate biopsy or in prostate secretions. These patients are otherwise free of any associated clinical signs or symptoms.

Seminal vesicles

Seminal vesicles can become inflamed or infected, and this condition is termed "seminal vesiculitis." These paired structures, which converge with the vas deferens to form the ampullary portion of the vas deferens, contribute a significant proportion of fluid to the ejaculate. **While seminal vesicles can become inflamed in isolation, seminal vesiculitis usually results from spread of infection or inflammation from other genitourinary sites such as the urethra, prostate, or bladder.** Patients with seminal vesiculitis often experience blood in the ejaculate (hematospermia), pelvic or perineal pain often made worse by ejaculation, and increased WBC levels in semen. **Underlying anatomical issues such as ejaculatory duct obstruction or seminal vesicle stones have been reported in association with seminal vesiculitis and may be the underlying cause in some cases.** Treatment with antibiotics directed to culture results (typically semen culture), anti-inflammatory therapy, and relief of any underlying anatomical anomalies are mainstay approaches to treating this relatively rare condition.

Vas deferens

Inflammation of the vas deferens, or vasitis, is a fairly rare clinical condition. Genitourinary tuberculosis, as well as more common genitourinary pathogens, should be considered as possible causative agents. On exam, patients with vasal inflammation will typically have vasal swelling and tenderness. Those patients with vasitis due to tuberculosis will sometimes have a "string of beads" configuration, with the "beads" representing mycobacterial tubercles. Treatment of vasitis should be directed toward the infecting organism, and anti-inflammatory therapy should also be considered. If more diffuse spermatic cord inflammation is noted, with involvement of more than just the vas deferens, a diagnosis of pseudosarcomatous proliferative funiculitis should be considered [5]. This condition is most commonly seen in spermatic cord ischemia or necrosis, and it is often initially misdiagnosed as sarcoma. The spermatic cord of an affected patient typically has areas of necrosis, inflammatory infiltrate, fibrin deposition, and spindle cell myofibroblastic proliferations. **In all types of vasal inflammation, lasting complications can potentially result, including vasal stenosis or vasal atresia. Vasal stenosis and atresia can lead to diminishment or outright loss of sperm contribution to the ejaculate from the affected side.**

Epididymis

Epididymitis is a fairly common clinical condition. Patients usually present with scrotal swelling and pain, which may be accompanied by systemic signs such as fever and elevated WBC count on complete blood count testing. Epididymal infection is the leading cause of epididymitis, although reflux of sterile urine to the epididymis has also been implicated as a cause. The latter condition, termed "reflux epididymitis," arises due to chemical irritation of the epididymis by urine. Patients with reflux epididymitis may have predisposing genitourinary anatomical abnormalities, such as anomalous insertion of the ejaculatory ducts into the prostatic urethra. Alternatively, some patients note a history of recent heavy lifting or Valsalva maneuver, which can force urine from the prostatic urethra in a retrograde fashion into the vas deferens and epididymis.

When infection is the cause of epididymitis, the underlying etiological organisms typically hinge on patient characteristics. More specifically, sexually active men are most commonly infected by *Chlamydia trachomatis*, and less commonly by *Neisseria gonorrhoeae*. Men who are not sexually active, who have had recent genitourinary instrumentation, and with anatomical abnormalities are more likely to have common uropathogens (gram-negative organisms such as *E. coli*, or the gram-positive *Enterococcus* species) as the root cause. **Acute epididymitis has clearly been linked to declines in sperm concentration and motility [1]. With therapy, improvement in these impaired semen parameters is typically observed. However, lasting declines can be seen when epididymal swelling and inflammation lead to outright epididymal obstruction on the affected side.** Treatment should be directed against the infecting organism determined by culture data, although co-infection with *Chlamydia trachomatis* and *Neisseria gonorrhoeae* should be considered in the case of sexually active men. Treatment should follow the recommendations for men with urethritis as detailed earlier in this chapter.

Orchitis

Orchitis can be caused by viral or bacterial infections. Viral infection most commonly results from hematogenous spread from other sites in the body, and bacterial orchitis more typically results from spread from other genitourinary structures such as the epididymis. While viral and bacterial orchitis share common symptoms, namely testicular swelling and tenderness, several important distinctions exist and will be detailed below.

Paramxyovirus, which causes mumps, is perhaps the most concerning viral cause of orchitis. Paramxyovirus (mumps) orchitis is seen in up to 20% of postpubertal men infected with the virus [3]. Testicular swelling and tenderness are generally seen about 4–6 days after the onset of parotid gland involvement. While the mumps vaccine has lessened the scope of this problem, historical data show that approximately 30% of patients with testicular involvement have bilateral involvement [3]. **Testicular atrophy is seen in 30–50% of men after mumps orchitis, and 25% of men with bilateral testicular involvement have resultant infertility.** Interestingly, coxsackie B virus is also capable of causing pathophysiological changes similar to those seen in paramyxovirus mumps orchitis.

Bacterial orchitis commonly results from bacterial infection spreading to the testicle from other structures in the genitourinary tract, namely the epididymis. A number of organisms, including *Chlamydia trachomatis, Neisseria gonorrhoeae,* gram-negative bacilli (*E. coli, Klebsiella* species, and *Pseudomonas* species) and gram-positive cocci (*Staphylococcus* species, *Streptococcus* species) are all capable of causing testicular infection. Patients often present with acute onset of scrotal swelling and pain, and may have fever and a reactive hydrocele. Antibiotic therapy should be tailored to the organisms growing in the urine, semen, prostate, or blood cultures, although initially, broad-spectrum antibiotics are often necessary while awaiting these results. **Occasionally, testicular infection may progress to abscess formation or testicular infarction, in which case abscess drainage or orchiectomy may be needed, respectively.** In these cases, scrotal ultrasound is usually helpful in determining the presence of an abscess and status of testicular blood flow.

Leukocytospermia

WBC infiltration is a hallmark immune system response to tissue infection or damage and is fundamental in restoring tissue back to normal health. Leukocytospermia, the condition characterized by elevated WBC levels in semen, can be seen in association with inflammation and/or infection of the various components of the male genitourinary tract. **Leukocytospermia is defined by the World Health Organization as $\geq 1 \times 10^6$ leukocytes/ml of semen.** The testis is an "immunologically privileged" site, and this status is maintained primarily by Sertoli cell tight

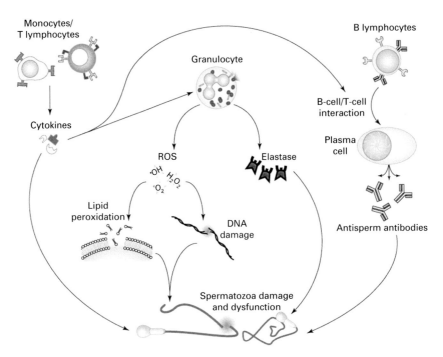

Figure 5.1 Paradigm for leukocyte subpopulation interaction in infertile men with leukocytospermia. Reproduced with permission from Lipshultz L, Howards S, Niederberger C, eds. *Infertility in the Male*, 4th edn (Cambridge, Cambridge University Press, 2009). ROS, reactive oxygen species.

junctions (forming the blood–testis barrier) that prevent WBCs from accessing the luminal aspect of the seminiferous tubules. Normal testicular tissue on biopsy is devoid of WBCs, affirming the notion that the blood–testis barrier helps prevent the immune system from generating a response to sperm antigens.

Early work by the insightful investigators Wolff and Anderson revealed that infertile men have higher concentrations of seminal leukocytes compared with fertile men [6]. More specifically, leukocytospermia has been shown to be associated with significant declines in total sperm number, sperm motility, sperm morphology, and various aspects of sperm function [1, 7]. While some studies suggest a potential beneficial role for seminal WBCs (scavengers of dead sperm, nonspecific defense mechanisms, etc.), the preponderance of medical literature at this time suggests that leukocytospermia overall is associated with negative effects on fertility [1].

Leukocytes initiate and maintain a complex series of steps in the immune system response; this is truly a highly orchestrated and regulated series of events involving cellular and humoral components (see Figure 5.1). More specifically, T lymphocytes, B lymphocytes, granulocytes, and macrophages are activated and proliferated to engage in specific roles in tissue defense. These roles include the release of cytokines, antibody production, the release of free radicals, and phago-cytosis of invading organisms and viruses. **These complex, defensive processes can also have very detrimental effects on sperm and anatomical components of the reproductive tract, leading to markedly impaired fertility** [1].

Cytokines are released by monocytes and lymphocytes and serve as the primary mode of communication within the immune system. Some cytokines promote a proinflammatory state, while others serve to resolve the inflammatory process. Tumor necrosis factor alpha, interleukin (IL)-1, and IL-6 are all proinflammatory cytokines. Elevation of several of these cytokines has been found to be associated with a decline in semen parameters and sperm function. For example, Naz and Kaplan reported that IL-6 elevations in infertile men were significantly correlated with detrimental effects on sperm number, motility, and penetration [8]. IL-4 and IL-10 are examples of cytokines that have anti-inflammatory effects, and several studies have shown that these anti-inflammatory cytokine levels are significantly lower in infertile men with and without leukocytospermia compared with normal fertile control patients [1]. One such study, by Omu *et al.*, revealed that IL-4 is lower in infertile men with leukocytospermia (with and without bacterial infection) and infertile men without leukocytospermia compared with fertile men [9]. **These studies collectively suggest that impaired ability to regulate the inflammatory process may hinder male fertility potential.**

Reactive oxygen species and oxidative stress

No discussion of leukocytospermia would be complete without a thoughtful discussion of reactive oxygen species (ROS). **ROS are also known as "free radical molecules" because they have an extra, unpaired electron.** Examples of ROS include the peroxyl radical, hydroxyl radical, superoxide anion, hydroxyl peroxide, and the hypochlorite radical. ROS molecules are highly unstable, and, as their name implies, they are reactive. ROS play a normal role in an array of routine physiological processes, including many aspects of reproductive function. For instance, ROS play a critical role in the process of sperm capacitation. **In the setting of inflammation and infection though, the normal endogenous antioxidant mechanisms (superoxide dismutase enzyme, catalase enzyme, and antioxidants) may be overwhelmed by increased ROS activity, leading to tissue damage.** Previous studies have documented the harmful effects of excess ROS in autoimmune, inflammatory, and infectious processes in other systems (i.e., cardiovascular), and now an abundance of studies have similarly confirmed their detrimental effects on male reproduction [1].

ROS are produced by two main populations of cells in the male reproductive tract, namely sperm and WBCs (specifically granulocytes). Interestingly, both immature and damaged spermatozoa have been shown to release higher levels of ROS than normal, mature spermatozoa [10]. The majority of ROS in the male reproductive tract though are produced by granulocytes. Indeed, granulocytes are responsible for the generation of approximately 1000 times higher levels of ROS than spermatozoa.

Numerous studies have demonstrated an association between elevated semen ROS levels and impaired male fertility [1]. ROS are capable of damaging the sperm membrane via lipid peroxidation, potentially resulting in sperm membrane dysfunction. Changes in the sperm membrane caused by ROS have been shown to subsequently lead to altered membrane composition, decreased sperm motility, and impaired sperm–egg fusion [11]. Elevated ROS levels can also cause sperm DNA damage as evidenced by increased sperm DNA fragmentation. These findings have been observed in studies comparing men with leukocytospermia to infertile men without leukocytospermia and healthy donors [12]. **Sperm DNA damage is widely acknowledged to decrease fertility potential, with possible detrimental effects on fertilization, pregnancy rates, and live births.**

Nitric oxide is another purported mediator of leukocyte damage to sperm. It can react with the superoxide anion free radical to create the peroxynitrite anion (ONOO), a highly reactive, cytotoxic molecule capable of causing significant cellular damage. The peroxynitrite molecule is believed to inhibit cellular aerobic respiration, leading to severe sperm damage and even death. The detrimental nitric oxide–peroxynitrite pathway has been demonstrated in sperm.

Antisperm antibodies

As mentioned previously in this chapter, the testis is an immunologically privileged site, and the immune system does not have exposure to spermatozoa due to the blood–testis barrier created by Sertoli cell tight junctions. **However, this immunologically privileged status can change with violation of the patient's blood–testis barrier, failure of immunosuppression, or inoculation of the host with sperm antigens.** The end result can be the formation of antisperm antibodies (ASA), which can have markedly negative effects on male fertility. **More specifically, ASA can lead to impaired sperm motility, agglutination of sperm, inhibition of cervical mucus penetration by sperm, and prevention of sperm–egg fusion.**

The humoral arm of the immune system is responsible for the production of ASA. Increased levels of IL-1, IL-2, and IL-6, combined with T-helper cell activity, can lead to B-cell transformation into plasma cells, which can then induce the production of specific ASA.

Several studies have shown an association between leukocytospermia and positive testing for ASA [1]. One study specifically showed a higher prevalence of ASA in leukocytospermia associated with microbial infection compared with leukocytospermia without microbial infection [9]. Both of these patient groups though had a higher prevalence of ASA compared with fertile controls.

Diagnostic testing for leukocytospermia, reactive oxygen species, and antisperm antibodies

Leukocytospermia diagnostic testing

As described above, leukocytospermia is defined by the World Health Organization as $\geq 1 \times 10^6$ leukocytes/ml of semen. **A key clinical consideration when contemplating a diagnosis of leukocytospermia is that "round cells" seen during routine semen testing can be mistakenly assumed to be WBCs. WBCs and immature sperm share similar visual features on phase contrast microscopy, and they can thus be mistaken for one another.** Indeed, immature sperm are a common finding in semen of infertile men. One study showed that when round cells are present, only a minority (35%) of affected men actually have leukocytospermia [13]. Immature sperm and leukocytes can both be present in semen samples, as they are not mutually exclusive. **The key message here is that the findings of round cells on phase microscopy alone are not sufficient to assign a diagnosis of leukocytospermia and additional studies are needed.**

More specific testing for seminal leukocytes includes Bryan–Leishman staining, peroxidase (Endtz) test, and monoclonal antibodies directed against leukocyte surface molecules. The Bryan–Leishman stain is not widely used, as it tends to overestimate lymphocytes and underestimate granulocytes in semen samples. The Endtz test stains peroxidase, and it thus only detects the granulocyte subpopulation of WBCs. The Endtz test is nonetheless useful because the majority of seminal leukocytes tend to be granulocytes. The best tests for detecting seminal leukocytes utilize immunohistochemical techniques. Antibodies directed against the WBC cell antigen CD45, also known as "leukocyte common antigen," will effectively detect not only granulocytes, but also macrophages and lymphocytes. Monoclonal antibodies can be more specifically directed against select subpopulations of WBCs (i.e. antibodies directed against CD15 specifically detect granulocytes). **In sum, immunohistochemical techniques provide the most accurate method of leukocyte identification and quantification compared with other available techniques.**

Reactive oxygen species diagnostic testing

The most commonly employed method of ROS detection involves chemiluminescence. With this technique, luminol, a molecular probe, emits light when it reacts with oxidative reaction end products. The light signal emitted during the reaction is detected by a machine called a luminometer, which provides a measure of ROS levels. The chemiluminescent assay must generally be performed within an hour of semen collection, as the oxidative activity of seminal oxidants declines over time.

Antisperm antibodies diagnostic testing

ASA can be detected via several different assays, the most prominent of which include the sperm mixed agglutination reaction (SpermMAR), the mixed agglutination reaction, and the Immunobead Rosette Test (IBT) (An overview of tests for ASA is available in [1], chapter 37, "Tests for antisperm antibodies.") **Of these tests, the most commonly used to detect ASA is the IBT; it is widely available and relatively inexpensive.** The IBT identifies both the class of antibodies binding to sperm and location on sperm where these antibodies are bound. Microscopic polyacrylamide beads covered with rabbit antibodies directed against human immunoglobins are used; these rabbit antibodies in turn bind to antibodies attached to the sperm surface. The immunoglobulins targeted may be whole human immunoglobulin or specific immunoglobulin classes (IgA, IgG, or IgM). The sperm and beads are incubated together, and the mixture is inspected microscopically to detect agglutination of sperm and beads. The substratification of specific immunoglobulin classes is relevant because IgAs are more harmful to sperm function than IgGs.

IBT may be performed in either a "direct method" or an "indirect method." In the "direct method," technicians directly assess for antibodies present on the patient's sperm surface. Immunobeads are incubated with the patient's sperm and subsequent inspection for sperm–immunobead binding is performed microscopically. This "direct method" IBT is the preferred test, but the patient must have an adequate number of motile sperm present in the ejaculated sample. The "indirect method" uses sperm from a donor who has previously been found to be negative for ASA using the "direct method." The donor's sperm and the patient's seminal fluid (his sperm have been removed) are incubated together, and ASA from the patient's seminal fluid is passively transferred to the donor's sperm. Incubation of this mixture with immunobeads is then undertaken and assessment of immunobead–sperm binding is performed.

While each laboratory has its own reference range for assays such as the IBT, positive results are generally noted when over 20% of the motile sperm have two or more attached immunobeads. In addition to recording the percentage of sperm positive for bead binding, the pattern of bead binding is also documented. Beads may be bound to the head, mid-piece, tail, or whole sperm regions. **The region of binding is an important consideration because it determines the impact of ASA on sperm function. Tail binding tends to interfere with sperm motility and forward progression, while head binding is more likely to result in impaired sperm–egg interaction (i.e., sperm–zona pellucida binding, sperm–oocyte fusion, and fertilization).** It is also believed that ASA may lead to alterations in normal sperm ion channel function, may promote premature induction of the acrosome reaction, and may induce complement-mediated sperm damage. (See [1], where chapter 16 addresses immunologic infertility and chapter 37 addresses tests for ASA, pp. 603–12. These chapters complement one another and both provide insight into the clinical significance of ASAs.)

Serum ASA testing to assess circulating ASAs is also possible. Circulating and seminal ASA are not necessarily correlated though and it appears that only ASA actually bound to sperm in semen have clinical relevance. At this time, it is unclear what pathophysiologic role, if any, circulating ASAs have. **Given the**

lack of clinical relevance of the results, testing for *circulating* ASA
is not recommended at this time.

Treatment options for immunologic infertility

Treatment of leukocytospermia

Several treatment options exist for leukocytospermia. The overall goal is to
resolve increased WBC levels and ameliorate the numerous harmful effects that
elevated levels of these cells bring to the male reproductive tract. The three major
classes of therapies are antibiotics, anti-inflammatory agents, and antihistamines,
which will be discussed below.

Antibiotics
A number of studies support the role of antibiotics in the treatment of leukocytospermia. The overriding aim of this therapy is to treat any underlying infection
present in the genitourinary tract, and thus facilitate resolution of the immune
system's inflammatory response.

A study by Omu *et al.* evaluated the effects of antibiotics on semen parameters, seminal antioxidant capacity, and ASA levels in men [14]. Three groups
of patients were studied: men with WBCs and bacteria in the semen; men with
WBCs but no bacteria in the semen; and fertile controls. The authors found
that at baseline, sperm concentration was significantly higher in the fertile
control group than in both groups with WBCs in the semen. Semen antioxidant
capacity was highest in the fertile control group, followed by patients with
leukocytospermia alone, and patients with both leukocytospermia and bacterospermia had the lowest semen antioxidant capacity. ASA were more prevalent in
the group with leukocytospermia and bacterospermia, compared with men with
leukocytospermia alone. Men with leukocytospermia underwent antibiotic
treatment based on culture sensitivities, and post-therapy the men in this
treatment group were found to have significantly improved sperm concentration and motility. Total semen antioxidant activity was also increased in this
group after treatment, but no differences in ASA levels were found after
therapy.

So what about empiric antibiotic therapy in the absence of bacterial infection? Yanushpolsky *et al.* performed a prospective, randomized, controlled
study of leukocytospermic men (and their partners) with unexplained infertility
and no evidence of genitourinary infection [15]. Some of the men were found
to have leukocytospermia, and these patients and their partners were then
randomized to: oral doxycycline 100 mg twice a day for 14 days; oral trimethoprim 160 mg/sulfamethoxazole 800 mg twice a day for 14 days; and no therapy.
The authors found that antibiotic treatment for leukocytospermia in the
absence of bacterial infection did *not* improve semen parameters to a statistically significant degree.

The preponderance of studies, as suggested by the two above, indicate that antibiotic therapy directed against specific organisms is potentially beneficial for semen quality. Antibiotic therapy in the absence of bacterospermia generally does not lead to improvement in semen parameters.

Anti-inflammatory agents

While anti-inflammatory agents are a mainstay treatment for leukocytospermia, the medical literature is surprisingly devoid of publications documenting clinical outcomes associated with their use in this setting [1]. Cyclooxygenase-2 inhibitors are anti-inflammatory agents that specifically inhibit prostaglandin production. A recent nonrandomized, prospective study assessing the use of cyclooxygenase-2 inhibitors in patients with leukocytospermia without evidence of concurrent bacterial infection supports this management strategy [16]. After 2 weeks of treatment with valdecoxib, patients with leukocytospermia were found to have a significant increase in sperm count, but not motility or morphology. The authors concluded that patients with leukocytospermia in the absence of concurrent bacterial infection may benefit from cyclooxygenase-2 inhibitor therapy. However, it is important to realize that this was a small study with a short duration of treatment.

Antihistamines

Antihistamine agents are drugs that stabilize mast cells, preventing their degranulation and release of proinflammatory mediators. A recent open-label, noncontrolled study of 55 men with leukocytospermia assessed the effects of 12 weeks of treatment with the second-generation antihistamine ketotifen [17]. Ketotifen therapy resulted in a statistically significant reduction in WBC concentration and improvement in sperm motility and morphology compared with pretreatment values. Interestingly, no difference in sperm concentration was observed. The authors concluded that ketotifen therapy has a role in the treatment of men with leukocytospermia, but the results should be interpreted cautiously as the study was nonrandomized, noncontrolled, and nonblinded. In sum, while there may be a role for antihistamine therapy for leukocytospermia, a paucity of studies have evaluated their effectiveness in this setting.

Treatment of reactive oxygen species

Lifestyle modification

A number of behaviors have been shown to lead to elevated ROS levels. As such, lifestyle modification is one means of potentially reducing elevated ROS concentration. While few studies actually document the effects of lifestyle modification, these interventions are generally easy to accomplish and should be considered [18]. Recommendations to decrease exposure to tobacco smoke and automotive exhaust are logical steps in terms of both reproductive and overall health. Systemic medical conditions, including cardiovascular disease, diabetes mellitus, infection, and cancer are all known to be associated with elevated levels of free radicals. While various studies show that optimization of these medical conditions will lead to improvement in reproductive potential it is not clear how much of this improvement is tied to optimization of elevated ROS levels.

Antioxidant therapy

A number of antioxidant supplements have been studied for their ability to scavenge free radicals and improve semen parameters. Although many of these studies lack ideal design, several do appear to show the beneficial effects of antioxidant therapy on male reproduction.

Vitamin C (ascorbic acid) is present in measurable amounts in both seminal fluid and sperm. Previous studies have shown that infertile men have reduced vitamin C concentration in their seminal plasma. A randomized, placebo-controlled trial of vitamin C supplementation in fertile men who were heavy smokers revealed that daily doses of 200 mg and 1000 mg resulted in improvements in sperm concentration, motility, and morphology compared with placebo [19].

Vitamin E (alpha-tocopherol) is present in the cell membrane and helps protect it from lipid peroxidation by free radicals. One study of men with low sperm motility showed that supplementation with vitamin E 300 mg/day resulted in decreased markers of membrane lipid peroxidation and increased motility over placebo [20]. Interestingly, pregnancies were recorded in 11 partners from the treatment group and none from the placebo arm over the 6-month study period. A double-blind, randomized, placebo-controlled study assessing effects of vitamin E 600 mg/day in men with high seminal levels of ROS resulted in improved zona pellucida binding [21].

Not all studies have demonstrated beneficial effects of vitamin C and vitamin E though. A randomized, placebo-controlled, double-blind study in men with asthenospermia and moderate oligoasthenospermia showed that 8 weeks of high-dose vitamin C and vitamin E did not result in improvement in semen parameters [22]. One potential criticism of this study was its length, as the treatment period was shorter than the length of a cycle of spermatogenesis. In sum, a number of studies assessing the effects of vitamin C and vitamin E therapy on semen parameters and sperm function have been conducted [1]. Yet, while these two antioxidant agents are among the most investigated in terms of reproductive effects, study results have generally been inconsistent. At this time, these two agents are both widely used clinically.

Coenzyme Q (CoQ_{10}) has been shown in a number of studies to have beneficial effects on male reproduction. CoQ_{10} is concentrated in the sperm mid-piece where it helps promote the mitochondrial respiratory chain, "recycles" vitamin E, and helps prevent membrane lipid peroxidation. In an uncontrolled trial, 6 months therapy with CoQ_{10} 400 mg/day was found to improve sperm motility when compared with baseline levels in men with idiopathic asthenospermia [23]. Another study investigating CoQ_{10} had *in vitro* and *in vivo* components. The *in vitro* component showed that incubation of sperm with CoQ_{10} led to increased sperm motility. The *in vivo* study revealed that oral supplementation with CoQ_{10} 60 mg/day resulted in improved fertilization rates during *in vitro* fertilization with intracytoplasmic sperm injection (IVF-ICSI) without concomitant changes in semen parameters [24].

Carnitine is another antioxidant utilized to help optimize male fertility. This agent works by removing acetyl-coenzyme A, the agent responsible for mitochondrial ROS, from the extracellular environment. A multicenter study showed improvement in sperm motility in men with asthenospermia, but subsequent randomized, controlled studies have failed to demonstrate beneficial effects on sperm motility or sperm concentration [25, 26]. Interestingly, carnitine is present in very high levels in the epididymis, approximately 2000 times higher than plasma levels. This fact has provided the rationale for many investigators to study the role of carnitine supplementation in infertile men.

While a number of studies report on the outcomes associated with various *in vivo* and *in vitro* antioxidant therapies, the literature overall is hampered by a lack of randomized, placebo-controlled, double-blind studies of sufficient duration of treatment and statistical power to provide meaningful clinical results. Moreover, pregnancy data, the most important outcome in fertility studies, is strikingly absent from the majority of these studies. As such, antioxidant therapies truly remain empiric in nature. Fortunately, the favorable side-effect profile, low cost, and ease of dosing of antioxidants makes their use as empiric therapy a reasonable option as infertile men try to optimize their reproductive potential.

Treatment of antisperm antibodies

Immune suppressive therapy

Tailored therapy specifically targeting suppression of ASA is unfortunately not available at this time. Less specific, systemic immune suppression is available, however, and this is the cornerstone of medical therapy for ASA. Corticosteroids provide suppression of both the humoral and cellular arms of the immune system. More precisely, steroid therapy acts to decrease cytokine release, suppress chemotaxis, and diminish antibody production, including ASA.

Results from clinical trials have shown somewhat encouraging results with immune suppressive therapy. Unfortunately, the majority of these studies suffer from a lack of nontreatment or placebo-controlled arms. Two randomized, controlled trials of corticosteroid therapy have been published. The first, a double-blind, placebo-controlled trial, involved high-dose, tapered regimens of methylprednisolone cyclically over a 3-month period of time. While the authors found a decline in sperm-associated IgG with treatment, there was no benefit for methylprednisolone therapy over placebo in semen parameters or men's subsequent fertility [27]. The second study involved subfertile men with circulating ASA. Prednisone 20 mg was administered two times per day on days 1–10 of the menstrual cycle for 9 months, followed by a washout period and crossover to the other arm [28]. This study revealed no difference in semen parameters, or circulating ASA levels, but semen ASA titers declined significantly. More importantly, the authors reported that men undergoing treatment were significantly more likely to achieve a pregnancy (31%) than those receiving placebo (9%). The differences in outcomes in the two above studies may result from a shorter, 3-month follow-up time for the first study, limiting the ability of those authors to fully detect effects of treatment (i.e., pregnancy). In sum, as suggested by the second study, there may be a role for the use of corticosteroids in the treatment of ASA. However, additional studies with proper design are needed to confirm these findings and more fully elucidate clinical outcomes. **Furthermore, prescribing physicians must be aware that corticosteroids can cause an array of adverse effects, including dyspepsia, acne, fluid retention, skin changes, weight gain, and aseptic necrosis. A discussion of these possible side-effects should be undertaken with the patient before initiating corticosteroid therapy.**

Sperm washing with intrauterine insemination or *in vitro* fertilization

Another approach to managing couples with male factor ASA is sperm washing with subsequent intrauterine insemination (IUI) or IVF. A variety of semen processing techniques is available, and they are most effective at removing unbound ASA from the seminal fluid. Removal of antibodies bound to sperm is more difficult, and methods involving the use of rapid dilutional washing, detergent washes, and enzymatic cleaning have all been employed with varying degrees of success. The overriding problem is that the more aggressive the treatment to dissociate the ASA–sperm bond, the greater the likelihood of resultant sperm damage.

Once the sperm preparation technique has been completed, IUI is a viable treatment option. No prospective, controlled trials gauging the effectiveness of IUI in the setting of ASA have been reported, and several retrospective studies based the diagnosis of "immunological infertility" on serum, not semen, ASA levels. Thus, it is very important for clinicians to closely examine inclusion criteria and patient characteristics when considering these studies. One study by Agarwal assessed sperm washing plus IUI in 45 couples with male seminal ASA [29]. He concluded that this approach diminishes the level of sperm-bound immunoglobulins and can improve the chance of conception, particularly in patients with >50% attachment of IgG, IgA, or both. **The key finding was that 33% of couples undergoing sperm washing and IUI for ASA achieved a pregnancy, versus only 19% of couples who underwent this procedure for other reasons.**

IVF is another therapeutic option that can be coupled with sperm-washing techniques. **Interestingly, fertilization and pregnancy rates are lower for IVF when the indication is immunologic infertility, compared with IVF for other reasons.** Additionally, the more extensive the percentage of sperm bound by ASA, the lower the success rates with IVF. The finding holds true for both IgA and IgG ASA. Pre-IVF treatment of men with prednisone has been studied and does not result in improved fertilization or pregnancy rates when compared with placebo [30].

IVF-ICSI affords patients with ASA the best odds of pregnancy based on available clinical research. With this approach, ASA-related difficulties with sperm transit through the female reproductive tract and sperm–oocyte interaction are bypassed as the processed sperm is injected directly into the oocyte. **IVF-ICSI fertilization and pregnancy rates are similar for couples with male ASA when compared with couples without male ASA** [30]. **A note of caution should be heeded though, as this study and others have revealed lower embryo quality in IVF-ICSI cycles where the man was ASA positive** [31]. This observation implies that ASA may affect post-fertilization embryo development in a deleterious fashion.

Conclusions

In this chapter, we have overviewed a breadth of immunological causes of male factor infertility. From a clinical standpoint, determining the site(s) of infection and/or inflammation is a key first step. Identifying causative organisms and providing appropriate medical treatment, including antibiotics and anti-inflammatory agents, are mainstays of therapy. The literature regarding leukocytospermia, ROS, and ASA suggest that all these immunological issues are associated with negative effects on male reproductive potential. While medical therapies for each of these problems are available, most published studies assessing their efficacy and outcomes suffer from suboptimal design. Hopefully, the future will offer enhanced understanding of the mechanisms involved in immunologic infertility, as well as therapies that more accurately target the underlying, specific reproductive tract pathophysiology at hand.

REFERENCES

[1] Lipshultz L, Howards S, Niederberger C, eds. *Infertility in the Male*, 4th edn (Cambridge, Cambridge University Press, 2009).
[2] Kohler TS, Yadven M, Manvar A, *et al.* The length of the male urethra. *Int Braz J Urol* 2008; **34**: 451–4.
[3] Krieger JN. Prostatitis, epididymitis, and orchitis. In *Mandell, Douglas, and Bennett's: Principles of Infectious Disease*, 6th edn, Mandell G, Bennett J, Dolin R, eds (Philadelphia, PA: Churchill-Livingstone, 2005), Section L, Chapter 105.
[4] Krieger JN, Nyberg L Jr, Nickel JC. NIH consensus definition and classification of prostatitis. *JAMA* 1999; **282**: 236–7.
[5] Michal M, Hes O, Kazakov DV. Mesothelial glandular structures within pseudosarcomatous proliferative funiculitis – a diagnostic pitfall: report of 17 cases. *Int J Surg Pathol* 2008; **16**: 48–56.
[6] Wolff H, Anderson DJ. Immunohistologic characterization and quantitation of leukocyte subpopulations in human semen. *Fertil Steril* 1988; **49**: 497–504.
[7] Wolff H, Politch JA, Martinez A, *et al.* Leukocytospermia is associated with poor semen quality. *Fertil Steril* 1990; **53**: 528.

[8] Naz RK, Kaplan P. Increased levels of interleukin-6 in seminal plasma of infertile men. *J Androl* 1994; **15**: 220.

[9] Omu AE, Al-Qattan F, Al-Abdul-Hadi FM, *et al.* Seminal immune response in infertile men with leukocytospermia: effect on antioxidant activity. *Eur J Obstet Gynecol Reprod Biol* 1999; **86**: 195–202.

[10] Gil-Guzman E, Ollero M, Lopez MC, *et al.* Differential production of reactive oxygen species by subsets of human spermatozoa at different stages of maturation. *Hum Reprod* 2001; **16**: 1922–30.

[11] Aitken RJ, Clarkson JS, Fishel S. Generation of reactive oxygen species, lipid peroxidation, and human sperm function. *Biol Reprod* 1989; **41**: 183.

[12] Saleh RA, Agarwal A, Kandirali E, *et al.* Leukocytospermia is associated with increased reactive oxygen species production by human spermatozoa. *Fertil Steril* 2002; **78**: 1215.

[13] Sigman M, Lopes L. The correlation between round cells and white blood cells in the semen. *J Urol* 1993; **149**: 1338–40.

[14] Omu AE, al-Othman S, Mohamad AS, *et al.* Antibiotic therapy for seminal infection. Effect on antioxidant activity and T-helper cytokines. *J Reprod Med* 1998; **43**: 857–64.

[15] Yanushpolsky EH, Politch JA, Hill JA, Anderson DJ. Antibiotic therapy and leukocytospermia: a prospective, randomized, controlled study. *Fertil Steril* 1995; **63**: 142–7.

[16] Lackner JE, Herwig R, Schmidbauer J, *et al.* Correlation of leukocytospermia with clinical infection and the positive effect of anti-inflammatory treatment on semen quality. *Fertil Steril* 2006; **86**: 601–5.

[17] Oliva A, Multigner L. Ketotifen improves sperm motility and sperm morphology in male patients with leukocytospermia and unexplained infertility. *Fertil Steril* 2006; **85**: 240–3.

[18] Patel SR, Sigman M. Antioxidant therapy in male infertility. *Urol Clin North Am* 2008; **35**: 319–30.

[19] Dawson EB, Harris WA, Teter MC, *et al.* Effect of ascorbic acid supplementation on the sperm quality of smokers. *Fertil Steril* 1992; **58**: 1034–9.

[20] Suleiman SA, Ali ME, Saki ZM, *et al.* Lipid peroxidation and human sperm motility: protective role of vitamin E. *J Androl* 1996; **17**: 530–7.

[21] Kessopoulou E, Powers HJ, Sharma KK, *et al.* A double-blind randomized placebo cross-over controlled trial using the antioxidant vitamin E to treat reactive oxygen species associated male infertility. *Fertil Steril* 1995; **64**: 825–31.

[22] Rolf C, Cooper TG, Yeung CH, *et al.* Antioxidant treatment of patients with asthenozoospermia or moderate oligoasthenozoospermia with high-dose vitamin C and vitamin E: a randomized, placebo-controlled, double-blind study. *Hum Reprod* 1999; **14**: 1028–33.

[23] Balercia G, Mosca F, Mantero F, *et al.* Coenzyme Q(10) supplementation in infertile men with idiopathic asthenozoospermia: an open uncontrolled pilot study. *Fertil Steril* 2004; **81**: 93–8.

[24] Lewin A, Lavon H. The effect of coenzyme Q on sperm motility and function. *Mol Aspects Med* 1997; **18**(Suppl.): S213–19.

[25] Costa M, Canale D, Filicori M, *et al.* L-carnitine in idiopathic asthenospermia: a multicenter study. Italian study group on carnitine and male infertility. *Andrologia* 1994; **26**: 155–9.

[26] Sigman M, Glass S, Campagnone J, *et al.* Carnitine for the treatment of idiopathic asthenospermia: a randomized, double-blind, placebo-controlled trial. *Fertil Steril* 2006; **85**: 1409–14.

[27] Haas GG, Manganiello P. A double-blind, placebo-controlled study of the use of methylprednisolone in infertile men with sperm-associated immunoglobulins. *Fertil Steril* 1987; **47**: 295–301.

[28] Hendry WF, Hughes L, Scammell G, *et al.* Comparison of prednisolone and placebo in subfertile men with antibodies to spermatozoa. *Lancet* 1990; **335**: 85–8.

[29] Agarwal A. Treatment of immunological infertility by sperm washing and intrauterine insemination. *Arch Androl* 1992; **29**: 207–13.

[30] Lahteenmaki A, Reima I, Hovatta O. Treatment of severe male immunological infertility by intracytoplasmic sperm injection. *Hum Reprod* 1995; **10**: 2824–8.

[31] Nagy ZP, Verheyen G, Liu J, *et al.* Results of 55 intracytoplasmic sperm injection cycles in the treatment of male-immunological infertility. *Hum Reprod* 1995; **10**: 1775–80.

Genetics of male reproductive medicine

Moshe Wald, MD

Introduction

Infertility, defined as the inability to conceive after 1 year of unprotected intercourse, affects up to 15% of all couples with a male factor being causative in 40–60% of those cases [1]. Between 15% and 30% of male factor infertility cases are believed to be caused by genetic abnormalities, with the incidence of identifiable genetic anomalies being 20-fold greater than that of the fertile population. Over the last decade, as the field of molecular genetics has advanced, the understanding of specific genetic defects that cause male factor infertility has also greatly expanded. However, applying this understanding to the clinical setting has only begun. Further, advances in assisted reproductive technology, specifically intracytoplasmic sperm injection (ICSI), allow couples to bypass significant male factor genetic abnormalities, potentially propagating genetic anomalies.

The goal of this chapter is to provide an overview of the most commonly known genetic aspects of male reproductive medicine with particular focus on clinical presentation and underlying genetic or molecular etiology. Specific treatment options will be discussed where appropriate.

Numerical chromosomal abnormalities

Aneuploidy, a genetic anomaly involving an abnormal number of chromosomes, is the most common chromosomal defect in infertile men and is particularly common in men with nonobstructive azoospermia [2]. Klinefelter syndrome (originally described in 1942 but not causatively linked to a genetic anomaly

An Introduction to Male Reproductive Medicine, ed. Craig Niederberger. Published by Cambridge University Press. © Cambridge University Press 2011.

until 1959) is the most common such abnormality in infertile men, with a prevalence of 5% in men with severe oligozoospermia and 13% in men who are azoospermic. Klinefelter syndrome has incomplete penetrance resulting in a phenotypic spectrum, though all patients have small testicles typically measuring between 8 and 10 cm^3 [3]. The classic triad of small and firm testes, azoospermia, and gynecomastia rarely presents [3]. Rather, on one end of the spectrum, there is near complete androgenic dysfunction presenting with failure of virilization at the expected time of puberty, gynecomastia, and a eunuchoid appearance (see [4], p. 252). At the other end of the spectrum, patients present only with infertility, as their low production of testosterone may be adequate to maintain other testosterone-dependent functions. Patients with Klinefelter syndrome routinely have elevated follicle-stimulating hormone consistent with their reduced level of spermatogenesis. Patients with this diagnosis also tend to have difficulty with expressive language learning, though this is also variable. The variety in presentation also explains the findings of a Danish registry study, which reported that only 10% of patients are diagnosed before puberty and only 25% of all cases are ever diagnosed. Genetically, the syndrome is defined by the presence of an extra X chromosome, which can quickly be identified by Barr body analysis, although a karyotype is required for definitive diagnosis. Other diagnostic tools include fluorescent in-situ hybridization, quantitative real-time polymerase chain reaction of the androgen receptor or array comparative genomic hybridization, all of which avoid the time-consuming cell culture necessary for karyotype analysis. Classic Klinefelter syndrome is 47,XXY and has a 1:500 prevalence, but examples of 48,XXYY and 48,XXXY as well as 49,XXXXY have been reported (prevalence 1:17,000 to 1:50,000 and 1:85,000 to 1:100,000, respectively) [5]. Patients with the rare forms of Klinefelter syndrome tend to present with more severe phenotypes, including characteristic facial and skeletal malformations and severe neurodevelopmental features. Both mosaic and nonmosaic forms of Klinefelter syndrome (47,XXY/46XY versus 47,XXY, respectively) exist, with mosaic forms having a higher degree of spermatogenesis. Of the two, the nonmosaic form is more common, although mosaic forms may occur in up to 22% of cases. Natural pregnancy is possible in some cases, more commonly in cases of mosaic Klinefelter. **Even in cases of Klinefelter syndrome with azoospermia, testicular sperm extraction has been reported to find spermatozoa suitable for ICSI in up to 69% of these patients, although some series report rates as low as 17%** [6]. Some researchers have noted that age is an independent predictor of success in surgical sperm extraction in patients with Klinefelter syndrome. In 2005, Okada *et al.* reported success rates as high as 81% for men age 25–29 and as low as 22% for men aged 40–44 [7]. This group also showed men younger than 35 had a significantly higher chance of success than men did over 35. A more recent study from 2009 suggested men younger than 32 had a better chance of successful surgical sperm retrieval [8]. Regardless of the exact age cutoff used, it appears that age is a strong independent predictor of success in surgical sperm retrieval in men with Klinefelter syndrome. While patients with this disease are able to achieve pregnancy using ICSI technology, they risk passing their genetic disease to their progeny. Live births of children that are 46,XX and 46,XY have been reported from fathers known to have Klinefelter syndrome. The question over preimplantation genetic testing is controversial given the slight increase in sex chromosomal (0.9%) and autosomal disomy (7.5%) in these patients. Interestingly, while the extra X chromosome may be maternal or paternal in origin, when the fathers of patients with Klinefelter syndrome are examined, the number of sex chromosome disomic sperm (24,XY) increases with age – from 10% higher in fathers in their 20s to 160% higher in fathers in their 50s. The supernumerary X has been reported to be paternal approximately half of the time and can only be due to meiosis I errors as meiosis II errors would result in either XXX or XYY children.

While the exact mechanism linking the known genetic defect in Klinefelter syndrome to the phenotypic presentation is unknown, current theories have centered on the concept of excess gene dosage. In 1961, Lyon theorized that one copy of the X chromosome is transcriptionally inactivated to allow equal dosages of the genes encoded on the X chromosome between males and females [9]. Additionally, it should be noted that because the X and Y chromosomes are hypothesized to have once been a homologous chromosome pair that have diverged through evolution, specific areas on the two chromosomes have retained pseudoautosomal regions that recombine during meiosis. Sequencing of these pseudoautosomal regions has suggested that they contain up to 28 genes and that as many as 10% of the genes encoded on the X chromosome in a normal male (46,XY) are expressed in the testes, indicating that X-chromosome inactivation is an incomplete process. These observations led to the hypothesis that the Klinefelter phenotype is due to excess gene product (assuming that more active gene copies correlates with more gene expression) from either the X-linked genes or from the genes located in the pseudoautosomal regions.

The second most frequent genetic aneuploidy associated with male infertility is 47,XYY syndrome (formerly Jacob's syndrome) originally reported in 1962 and now known to have an incidence of 1:1000 live births [10]. Mosaic forms of the disease (46,XY/47,XXY) have also been reported. Two mechanisms have been proposed to explain the supernumerary chromosome – either paternal non-disjunction at meiosis II (84%) or a post-zygotic mitotic error (16%). Phenotypically, these men are normal, though reports of increased height and behavioral problems have been noted. Natural pregnancy is not uncommon in men with this condition but severe oligospermia or even azoospermia related to maturation arrest or Sertoli-only syndrome has been reported [11]. The majority of these men have normal spermatogenesis with the extra Y chromosome appearing to be lost in meiosis (though debate on whether this is an active or a random process remains) as less than 1% of sperm are 24,XY or 24,YY [11].

Mixed gonadal dysgenesis (45,X/46,XY) is another chromosomal anomaly that leads to infertility in male patients. In 60% of cases, clinical presentation includes sexual ambiguity, a streak ovary, and one testis [12]. Approximately

30% are phenotypically female but are sexually infantile with bilateral streak ovaries [12]. The least common presentation (~10%) are phenotypic males with bilaterally descended testicles [12]. On infertility evaluation, this latter group presents with azoospermia and elevated gonadotropins. Karyotype examination can reveal a ring Y chromosome, which can form after a break in the Y chromosome with loss of genetic information before subsequent re-fusing. The ring Y anomaly can cause a lag in anaphase leading to 45,X cell. Importantly, testicular biopsy will reveal Sertoli cell-only syndrome with normal Leydig cells and these dysgenetic gonads are at increased risk of developing gonadoblastoma or dysgerminoma.

Another chromosomal anomaly that can lead to male infertility is a chromosomal translocation or inversion. A translocation occurs when a segment of two separate chromosomes is exchanged. An inversion is a break in one chromosome and subsequent reverse orientation of that same segment of chromosome. The most common translocation is a Robertsonian translocation, which is the fusion of two acrocentric chromosomes, occurring in 0.8% of infertile men [3]. Chromosomes 13, 14, 15, 21, and 22 are known to be susceptible to fertility affecting translocations. Most such translocations are balanced, whereby no genetic material is lost, so that the patient is often clinically normal and presents with otherwise unexplained oligospermia. Patients with such translocations are at risk of passing their chromosomal defect to their offspring.

Understanding the anomalies of chromosomal numbers is important to any practicing specialist in male infertility as the correct diagnosis facilitates proper management of these common clinical problems.

Y-chromosomal anomalies

The Y chromosome is of particular interest in cases of male infertility. This chromosome is approximately 60 million base pairs long and can be functionally divided into three sections. Two pseudoautosomal regions are located at the distal tips of each arm of the chromosome and are involved in recombination with similar regions on the X chromosome. The function of the second region, the heterochromatic region, is currently unknown. The last region is the euchromatic region, which contains numerous genes required for sperm production. Anomalies of Yq, the long arm of the Y chromosome, have been correlated with male infertility for over 30 years. Eight palindromic sequences exist in the euchromatic portion of Yq, each containing segments that are repeated at least twice and may have another copy elsewhere on the Y chromosome. This arrangement is theorized to assist in genomic self-correction as, unlike the autosomal chromosomes, only one copy of the Y chromosome exists. However, the presence of these homologous palindromic sequences increases the chance of self-recombination with resultant deletion of genetic material.

The specific region on Yq related to infertility is termed the azoospermia factor area (AZF, Yq11) and has been divided into three subdivisions (a, b, c) based on their effect on spermatogenesis and testicular histology (OMIM 415000) [13]. **Deletions in the AZF region are common in both oligospermic (8%) and azoospermic (15%) patients.** In men with sperm density lower than 5 million/ml, up to 5% have the Y chromosome microdeletion. De novo mutations in this region are most common, likely due to the significant number of palindromic DNA sequences present, which allow intrachromosomal recombination with subsequent deletion of genetic information [14]. To understand the effect of either individual or combined deletions of this chromosome on fertility, it is best to examine each area individually.

AZFa spans 400–600 kb of DNA and is located on the proximal portion of the long arm of chromosome Y close to the centromere [15]. Up to 1% of men with nonobstructive azoospermia have deletion of this region [4]. **Complete deletions of the AZFa region are associated with azoospermia whereas partial deletions of this region are associated with marginal spermatogenesis** [16]. This observation can be understood by examining the genes located in this region, specifically *USP9Y* and *DBY* [17]. *DBY* (dead box on Y; OMIM 400010, Yq11) encodes an ATP-dependent RNA helicase and is involved in the development of premeiotic germ cells. Studies have shown that men with azoospermia often have a reduction in the quantity of *DBY* transcript, suggesting this gene plays a key role in spermatogenesis. Deletion of *USP9Y* (ubiquitin-specific protease 9, chromosome Y; OMIM 400005, Yq11.2) has been associated with oligospermia or oliogoasthenozoospermia suggesting that while it plays a role in spermatogenesis, it is less critical than the role played by *DBY*. Additionally, deletion of *USP9Y* is known to have been naturally transmitted to progeny in at least two families, suggesting that the protein is not required for sperm–egg interaction. Deletion of this region is theorized to occur by recombination of two retroviral elements (HER-V15yq1 and HERV15yq2) that flank the genomic material of importance. Histologically, complete deletion of this region is associated with germ cell aplasia or Sertoli cell-only histology (type 1) whereas partial deletions of this region result in mixed histology [3]. No reports exist of successful surgical sperm retrieval in patients with complete deletion of this region.

Clinically, region AZFb is similar to AZFa in that complete deletions of this region are associated with very little, if any, chance of finding ejaculated sperm whereas ejaculated sperm can be found in cases of partial deletions of this region [16]. AZFb is a longer section of Yq containing between 1 and 3 Mb of DNA and is located on the distal end of the long arm of chromosome Y extending 1.5 Mb into the AZFc region, though debate still exists over whether the AZFb region is distinct from the AZFc region. This region is also home to two essential genes for fertility, *RBMY* (RNA binding motif on the Y; OMIM 400006, Yq11.23) and *PRY* (translation–initiation factor 1A, Y isoform; OMIM 400019, Yq11.223). *RBMY* encodes the RNA-binding protein found in spermatogonia, spermatocytes, and round spermatids [18]. The *PRY* gene is involved in apoptosis regulation [18]. AZFb lies between palindrome P5 and P1 in a region with a significant number of homologous zones allowing for recombination and subsequent deletions of varying lengths of DNA to occur. Deletion of AZFb, AZFc, and combination deletion of AZFb/c are a result of the recombination of these homologous regions [19]. Interestingly, a deletion of all regions of AZFb except for the *RBMY* and *PRY* is associated with the presence of sperm. Histologically, complete deletion of AZFb presents with maturation arrest whereas partial deletion presents with mixed histology [3]. **Microdeletions of either the entire AZFa or AZFb regions of the Y chromosome were reported to be associated with exceptionally poor prognosis for successful sperm retrieval.** Men with nonobstructive azoospermia and AZF b/c deletions (as a result of a recombination error) also have a very poor chance of successful surgical sperm retrieval [16].

AZFc is the largest of the regions of interest, containing approximately 3.5 Mb of DNA and located on the distal part of Yq [15]. **AZFc deletions, the most common of the three regions affected, have the least impact on spermatogenesis. It has been reported that sperm could be found in the ejaculate of 38% of men with isolated AZFc deletions, and that surgical sperm retrieval via testicular sperm extraction or diagnostic testicular biopsy was successful in 56–67% of azoospermic men with isolated AZFc deletions** [20]. These patients were reported to have a quantitative but not qualitative deficiency in their sperm. Interestingly, deletions in the AZFc region appear to vary greatly with geographic location, complicating analysis of partial deletions of this region. As a result, numerous studies have reported varying correlations with partial deletion and spermatogenesis [2]. Structurally, this region contains numerous repeating blocks of DNA, termed amplicons, which are organized into sequence families. This format allows for significant genetic variation. One gene of specific interest to fertility is located in this region, *DAZ* (deleted in azoospermia; OMIM 400003, Yq11). *DAZ* codes for germ cell specific RNA-binding proteins as well as being involved in the maintenance of primordial germ cell population via meiosis. Mutations in this specific gene are found in 13% of cases of male infertility and up to 15% of men with azoospermia have complete deletion of this gene [15]. Seven copies of the gene exist, spanning 380 kb of DNA on Yq and four of these copies exist as inverted pair clusters with only single nucleotide polymorphisms. Deletion of as few as two of the *DAZ* genes have been linked to reduced spermatogenesis [15].

Other genes of potential interest have been identified in this region, including *CDY1* (chromodomain Y1; OMIM 400016, Yq11.23) and *BPY2* (basic protein Y2; OMIM 400016, Yq11). Although their function is unknown, the observation that their expression is limited to the testis makes them worthy of future research [15]. Histologically, deletions of this region are associated with hypospermatogenesis and Sertoli-cell only syndrome (type II) [3]. This is an important distinction because surgical sperm retrieval in azoospermic patients with AZFc deletion is successful in up to 55% of cases [16]. Combined with those patients with only severe oligospermia, only 19% of patients with isolated AZFc deletion have no sperm available for assisted reproductive techniques (see [4], p. 255). The success of assisted reproductive techniques to use retrieved sperm in patients with AZFc deletions raises the question of preimplantation genetic screening given that it is possible to select only those 24,X sperm for use, thus eliminating the risk of passing the condition on to the next generation.

Overall, the Y chromosome remains one of the most interesting areas of genetic research in male infertility and certainly, the best developed from a clinical standpoint. While technology today does not allow us to "cure" patients with Y-chromosomal anomalies, the information we learn from Y-chromosomal microdeletion analysis does allow us to guide clinical decision-making. It also assists many of these patients to father children through assisted reproduction techniques. In doing this, they have a clearer understanding of the genetic risks to their progeny.

X-chromosomal anomalies

In the male patient, the X chromosome is active in mitotically dividing cells but was classically thought to become translationally inactivated during early meiosis by a process called meiotic sex chromosome inactivation. Recent evidence, however, suggests that this inactivation process is incomplete and that at least some multicopy genes do continue to be expressed postmeiotically. Additionally, given that men only have one copy of the X chromosome, which is of maternal origin, women can be silent carriers of abnormal recessive X-linked male fertility genes, which will only become clinically apparent when expressed in the male son of such a carrier. These insights, combined with the need to identify the causes of approximately 75% of idiopathic male infertility have led researchers to explore the X chromosome for important genes in male fertility.

An example of an X-chromosome-linked single gene mutation, which can result in male infertility, is Kallmann syndrome. Kallmann syndrome, with an incidence of 1:30,000 live births, has both X-linked and autosomal components [3]. The X-linked form of this disease is most common, resulting from deletion of the *KAL1* gene (OMIM 308700) at Xp22.3 coding for anosmin 1, which is a neural cell adhesion protein, resulting in failure of migration of gonadotropin-releasing hormone (GnRH) neurons to the preoptic area of the hypothalamus. Autosomal forms include a dominant form of the disease linked to deletion of the gene *KAL2* (or fibroblast growth factor receptor 1 gene; OMIM 147950, 8p11.2–8p11.1), which is causative in 20% of cases of Kallmann syndrome, a recessive form of the disease linked to gene *KAL3* (OMIM 244200, 20p13) caused by a mutation in the G protein-coupled prokineticin receptor-2 gene (*PROKR2*) and associated with 10% of cases of Kallmann syndrome. **Clinical presentation includes central hypogonadism, anosmia, small testes, with rare renal agenesis, cleft lip, deafness, and asymmetry of the cranium and face** (see [4], p. 202). The testicular pathology varies from Sertoli cell-only syndrome to focal areas of spermatogenesis [3]. Clinical identification of this syndrome is important because medical management with gonadotropin replacement results in ejaculated sperm and normal pregnancies in up to 80% of patients.

Hypogonadotropic hypogonadism without anosmia is often termed idiopathic hypogonadotropic hypogonadism and can result from any one of numerous known genetic anomalies. One X-chromosome-linked example is a defect in *DAX1* (OMIM 300473, Xp21.3–21.2), a gene that encodes a group of steroid receptors required for the development of the hypothalamus, pituitary, adrenal glands, and gonads. The role this gene plays in adrenal gland development explains why these patients present with congenital adrenal hypoplasia and are at risk of severe electrolyte problems early in life. Other genetic causes of idiopathic hypogonadotropic hypogonadism include defects in the *GRHR* (the GnRH receptor gene, OMIM 138850, 4p21.2) or *PC1* (prohormone convertase 1 gene, OMIM 162150, 5q15–q21). Loss of function of the GnRH receptor (which is a G coupled calcium-dependent receptor) via any one of almost a dozen known deficiencies creates a functional disconnect between the hypothalamus and the pituitary with resulting decreased gonadotropin release. *PC1* encodes a protein, convertase 1, which is a serine endoprotease involved in secretion of GnRH by the hypothalamus. In addition to idiopathic hypogonadotropic hypogonadism, *PC1* deletion is associated with obesity and diabetes (see [4], p. 266).

The androgen receptor gene is also located on the X chromosome and has implications for male fertility. Its role will be discussed below in the section summarizing all chromosomal anomalies of androgen metabolism and signaling. **In summary, the X chromosome plays a vital role in male fertility and numerous genes have been identified, which with further research may help explain idiopathic male infertility.**

Chromosomal anomalies of androgen metabolism and signaling

The understanding of the role androgens play in male reproduction has significantly advanced since Dr. Brown-Séquard's pioneering work in 1889, and much information has been obtained regarding androgen biosynthesis and receptor signaling pathways. Genetic anomalies at any point in these processes can have significant clinical implications. Thus, known genetic anomalies at different steps of androgen biosynthesis and receptor signaling pathways will be described, with attention to their clinical presentation.

The rate-limiting step in the synthesis of androgen is the process of transferring cholesterol from the outer to the inner mitochondrial membrane, which is facilitated by the steroidogenic acute regulatory protein (StAR). Genetic anomalies of this step (including single nucleotide transversions) have been identified and present as congenital lipoid adrenal hyperplasia (OMIM 600617, 8p11.2). Other anomalies of the steroid synthesis pathway have been identified and negatively impact fertility, including deficiency of 17beta-hydroxysteroid dehydrogenase type 3 (phenotypic females who develop male secondary sex characteristics at puberty; OMIM 264300, 9q22) and deficiency of testicular 17,20-desmolase (male pseudohermaphroditism; OMIM 309150, chromosome unknown).

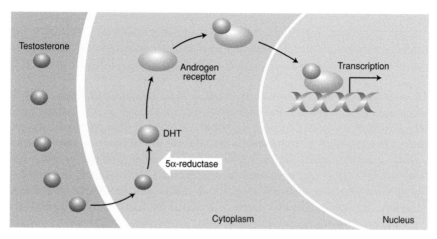

Figure 6.1 Testosterone enters the cell and is reduced to 5α-dihydrotestosterone (DHT) by 5α-reductase. DHT binds to the androgen receptor, and the complex moves into the nucleus, where transcription control of androgen-dependent genes occurs. Reproduced with permission from Malagarie-Cazenave S *et al.* Sphingolipid signaling: molecular basis and role in TNF-α-induced cell death. *Exp Rev Mol Med* 2002; 4: 1–15. Cambridge University Press.

Once synthesized, androgens are transported to their target tissue via the blood-stream where the majority (over 98%) of serum testosterone is bound to sex hormone binding globulin and albumin and exists in equilibrium with the 1–2% that is free and biologically active. **The role of sex hormone binding globulin is not limited to merely passively binding testosterone in the serum, rather, it plays an important role in spermatogenesis by controlling the concentration of androgens in the testis** (OMIM 182205, 17p13–p12). One study investigating polymorphisms in the gene for sex hormone binding globulin has associated shorter sex hormone binding globulin genes with increased levels of spermatogenesis, though this observation and any negative effect of longer sex hormone binding globulin genes on spermatogenesis will need further clarification [21].

Testosterone, like all steroids, is lipophilic and freely diffuses through the cell membrane to the cytoplasm where the androgen receptor is located. In some cells, testosterone is converted to 5α-dihydrotesterone by 5α-reductase before affecting the cell (Figure 6.1). 5-Alpha-dihydrotesterone is particularly important in the embryological development of the prostate, external male genitalia, and urethra. **Genetic anomalies of the 5-alpha reductase type 2 gene (OMIM 607306, 2p23) results in a 46,XY intersex condition.** Of note, 5-alpha reductase type 1 is not expressed during fetal development so is not related to developmental anomalies. This condition, previously known as pseudovaginal perineoscrotal hypospadia, more commonly creates a spectrum of disease ranging from full female to full male phenotypes at birth. All these patients, however, develop male secondary sex characteristics at puberty due to the increase in testosterone production from the testicles. Over 50 specific anomalies of this gene have been reported, most commonly missense mutations, but ranging from premature stop codons to complete deletions. Proper identification of this disease is important for family counseling, as over 50% of patients who are raised as females switch to a male gender at puberty.

Once testosterone reaches a target cell, it must interact with its receptor to cause an effect. Details of the androgen receptor are beyond the scope of this chapter and are well reviewed in other texts. However, in summary, the receptor must bind to testosterone, translocate to the nucleus, interact with DNA, and allow transcription of downstream genes (see [4], p. 257). The importance of this process cannot be understated, as a properly functioning receptor is vital for male embryologic development, regulation of the epididymis and seminal vesicles in the adult, and control of spermatogenesis via interaction with the Sertoli cell [4].

The incidence of androgen receptor gene mutations is estimated at 1:60,000 live births with the severity of the clinical phenotype inversely correlating with the degree of receptor function [3]. As a result, the phenotype ranges from normal-appearing females with testicles (complete androgen insensitivity) to normal-appearing but infertile males. The wide clinical spectrum of androgen receptor gene mutations is evident by the numerous names given to it, ranging from descriptive terminology such as complete, partial, or minimal androgen insensitivity syndrome to the eponyms such as Kennedy, Reifenstein, Lub, and Rosewater's diseases (see [4], p. 258).

Genetically, the androgen receptor is located on the X chromosome at Xq11–12 and approximately 800 mutations have been described (OMIM 313700). A web-based international database exists that lists known mutations and their associated phenotypes (http://androgendb.mcgill.ca/). The gene that codes for the androgen receptor protein includes four sections and eight exons: a transactivation domain (exon 1), a well-conserved DNA-binding domain (exons 2 and 3), hinge section, and ligand-binding domain (exons 4–8). Located in the transactivation domain is a series of CAG repeats whose length has been reported to be associated with sperm density, though controversy over this hypothesis exists.

Complete androgen insensitivity, or testicular feminization, occurs in 1:20,000 live births and presents clinically as a normal-appearing female with testicles present, but with a karyotype of 46,XY. While it has been described since 1953, case reports exist before that time and modern historians have gone so far as to theorize that both Joan of Arc and Queen Elizabeth I had the disease, though such theories obviously lack definitive proof. Of note, the prevalence of the disease rises dramatically to 1.4% in the population of females with inguinal hernias. Clinically, these patients are phenotypically normal females, including normal breast development and height (which differentiates them from Swyer's syndrome or complete gonadal dysgenesis, which lacks those two latter features) who have blind-ending vaginas and a decreased degree of axillary and pubic hair. The testicles continue to produce testosterone and due to a lack of feedback, elevated levels of testosterone are not uncommon [22]. As up to 5% of all dysgerminomas occur in patients with complete androgen insensitivity or gonadal dysgenesis, it is recommended to remove the testicles in these patients after puberty.

Partial androgen insensitivity syndrome, originally described by Reifenstein, ranges clinically from isolated hypospadias to clitoromegaly. Infertility in these patients can result from the failure of male development. Lastly, minimal androgen insensitivity syndrome has been described, in which phenotypic males present with oligospermia and normal testosterone levels but elevated luteinizing hormone levels, suggesting a poorly functioning androgen receptor [22].

Kennedy's syndrome, or X-linked spinal and bulbar muscular atrophy (OMIM 313700.0014), deserves specific mention because of the unique manner of presentation. These rare patients (estimated 1:40,000) develop a slowly progressive adult onset (average age of presentation is mid-40s) form of bulbar and extremity muscle weakness; often initially presenting with muscle cramps but leading to extremity muscle weakness and, eventually, bulbar signs such as dysarthria and dysphagia. While the disease syndrome was described in 1968, the etiology was not described until 1991. The etiology is an increase in the CAG repeat number found in exon 1 of the androgen receptor, normally coding for the transactivation domain [23]. While the normal number of CAG repeats varies between 11 and 35, patients with Kennedy's syndrome have between 40 and 62 total repeats, with a greater number of repeats correlating with disease severity. From an endocrine standpoint, gynecomastia, reduced fertility (azoospermia or oligozoospermia), testicular hypotrophy, and normal or elevated testosterone levels with elevated luteinizing hormone are commonly present and consistent with a partial androgen sensitivity defect [23]. As with the muscle-related signs, the endocrine manifestations tend to develop later in life, allowing the majority of these patients to be fertile early in life, though many become azoospermic as they age [23]. During genetic counseling of patients, especially when considering assisted reproductive techniques, it is important to consider the phenomenon of anticipation that subsequent generations inherit larger repeat sequences than the father, with potential worse disease phenotype [3].

Other single gene mutations

Certain forms of male factor infertility can be attributed to a single gene mutation. One such example is the translocation of the *SRY* gene associated with the 46,XX male syndrome (formerly known as de la Chapelle syndrome, OMIM 400045). Up to 10% of 46,XX true hermaphrodites are SRY+. The *SRY* gene is normally located on the short arm of the Y chromosome at Yp11.3 and encodes a highly conserved DNA-binding motif that alters the three-dimensional structure of DNA, allowing specific genes to be targeted. In this case, targeted genes cause differentiation of the Sertoli cells, which is the earliest recognizable step in male differentiation. Clinical presentation of these men can range from ambiguous genitalia to normal male phenotype with azoospermia.

A second single gene mutation, which can result in male factor infertility, is an anomaly in the *CFTR* (cystic fibrosis transmembrane conductance regulator) gene located on chromosome 7q31.2, which encodes a cyclic adenosine monophosphate regulated chloride channel involved in maintaining the viscosity of epithelial secretions (OMIM 602421). Clinically, these patients present with obstructive azoospermia and nonpalpable vas deferens bilaterally, though only 60–90% of patients who present with congenital bilateral absence of the vas deferens (CBAVD) have a defect in the *CFTR* gene [17]. A second as yet unidentified genetic anomaly involved in mesonephric duct differentiation is currently believed to be responsible for the remainder of CBAVD cases (OMIM 277180) [4]. As neither mutation affects spermatogenesis, the physical exam is otherwise benign, though a transrectal ultrasound will likely show unusual seminal vesicles, which can range from atrophic to dilated and cystic. Recent evidence has suggested that the *CFTR* gene mutation may also directly affect sperm production and fertilizing capacity, though this requires further investigation. These patients have a low volume, low fructose, and low pH ejaculate, consistent with acidic prostatic secretions that predominate.

Up to 1 in 20 people of northern European descent is a carrier of a dysfunctional cystic fibrosis gene, with over 1200 different mutations currently identified [24]. The most common mutation is a 3 base pair deletion termed deltaF508, which results in deletion of a phenylalanine residue and is responsible for 60–70% of cases of CBAVD. The resulting modification of the protein product is believed to cause disease by altering the natural processing of the protein product, resulting in altered retention of the mis-folded mutant product in the endoplasmic reticulum. Some mutations are more severe than others are and the exact clinical presentation of a patient with cystic fibrosis will depend on details of their mutations. Men homozygous for two "mild" mutations may only present with CBAVD, whereas men homozygous for more severe mutations will have pulmonary and intestinal symptoms as well as infertility [3]. It has been theorized that idiopathic CBAVD is actually one extreme of the spectrum of cystic fibrosis and, in fact, cases of CBAVD or idiopathic epididymal obstruction are associated with an increased risk of *CFTR* mutation.

While point mutations are the most common cause of *CFTR* mutations, another common anomaly is a variation in the polythymidine tract of the splicing region of intron 8. A decrease to only five thymidines in this thymidine tract has been associated with up to a 50% reduction in *CFTR* mRNA.

Men with CBAVD and *a known CFTR* gene mutation do not need to be screened for renal anomalies. However, up to 10% of patients with CBAVD and *no CFTR* gene identified will be found to have renal anomalies, including agenesis and hypoplasia, indicating that screening in this subpopulation is required [25]. **Men with CBAVD should also be counseled to discuss their diagnosis with their family members given the possibility that they may either have the disease or are carriers.** Surgical sperm retrieval followed by

ICSI bypasses the anatomical problem created in these patients though risks passing on the genetic anomaly to the patient's progeny unless screening is conducted.

A third genetic defect, which can present as male factor infertility, is persistent Müllerian duct syndrome. These patients have normal external and internal male genitalia as well as a fully developed uterus, cervix, upper two-thirds of the vagina, and fallopian tubes. Male patients with this disease present in one of two ways. The first is with hernia uteri inguinalis, characterized by a descended testis and herniation of the uterus and ipsilateral fallopian tube into the inguinal canal. The second is crossed testicular ectopia, characterized by herniation of both testes and the entire uterus and both fallopian tubes. The etiology of this condition is related to failure of normal male embryological differentiation. Up to the seventh week of gestation, the fetus contains both Müllerian and Wolffian structures, but soon after the testes differentiate, the fetal Sertoli cells secrete Müllerian inhibiting substance (or anti-Müllerian hormone) leading to normal male differentiation. The failure of Müllerian structures to involute is believed to be due to a failure of the body to produce, properly time the release of, or recognize Müllerian inhibiting substance. Defects in both the Müllerian inhibiting substance gene (type 1, OMIM 261550, 19p13.3–13.2) and its receptor gene (type 2, OMIM 261550, 12q13) have been described. The condition has been described as both an X-linked and autosomal dominant pattern, though the location of the X-chromosome-related genetic anomaly is unknown [3]. Any undescended testicle in these men should be treated like any other, as the risk of malignant transformation appears to be similar. Care must also be exercised during surgical correction of any hernia, as these men are otherwise fertile.

Epigenetics

Epigenetics is the study of inherited genetic traits that are not due to changes in the underlying DNA sequence, thus the addition of the prefix "epi" (Greek for above or over) to the root word "genetics." **Epigenetic changes include covalently attached molecules such as methylation and acetylation as well as closely associated proteins such as histones in somatic cells and both histones and protamines in sperm. Numerous examples of defects in this process, which can negatively affect spermatogenesis have been defined.** The importance of methylation control has been demonstrated in both *Caenorhabditis elegans* and mouse models where loss of the genes coding for H3K4me demethylase and JmjC domain containing histone demethylase 2A respectively have resulted in infertility. Unfortunately, studies to date examining the methylation pattern of infertile men have found no abnormalities. The histone acetylation status of specific lysine residues is also tightly controlled during spermatogenesis where histone acetylation is associated with chromatin relaxation and gene transcription and histone de-acetylation is associated with gene silencing.

Defects in this process have resulted in defective spermatogenesis in mouse models and their role in humans is under investigation.

During spermatogenesis, sperm DNA undergoes significant changes in how it is packaged, including the exchange of most histones for one of two protamines (P1 or P2), which are proteins that tightly bind to DNA forming toroids. The use of toroids increases the level of DNA compaction, which is key to genome transport. The histone for protamine exchange is not complete, however, with up to 15% of histones remaining. Interestingly, the conversion of histones to protamines requires an intermediate step whereby transitional proteins are inserted. Mouse studies have shown that disruption of the genes responsible for these transitional proteins produces infertile mice.

While it was originally believed that the small percentage of remaining histones was simply the result of random incomplete exchange, evidence that histones are not replaced at specific locations has recently emerged. One study showed that histones were specifically enriched at promoters of specific imprinted genes, including *YBX2* involved in spermatogenesis (OMIM 611447, 17p13.1–p11.2). The role of the two variants of protamines is also being investigated. It is known that men with unequal P1/P2 ratios have decreased sperm quality and it is theorized that such abnormal ratios may be associated with gene imprinting. A single nucleotide polymorphism in the gene for P1, G197T, has been identified and is associated with DNA fragmentation and teratozoospermia (OMIM 182880, 16p13.3).

The significant epigenetic changes that occur to sperm DNA during spermatogenesis create numerous opportunities for errors to appear and propagate with negative impact on fertility. Ongoing research will clarify the extent of this phenomenon and its role in male factor infertility.

DNA repair and recombination errors

DNA damage is a common event with some sources estimating that between 1000 and 1,000,000 lesions per cell occur daily out of an estimated 3 billion base pairs. Mutations in the genes responsible for repairing this damage (e.g., *PMS2* [OMIM 600259, 7p22] and *Mlh1* [OMIM 120436, 3p21.3]) are associated with malignancies such as colon cancer, retinoblastoma, and melanoma [3]. Further, it is known that mice deficient in these genes are also infertile due to maturation arrest likely due to abnormal chromosome synapsis during meiosis. Evidence from humans with histological maturation arrest and Sertoli cell-only syndrome has shown an association between these syndromes and increased levels of damaged DNA, suggestive of an inability to repair DNA [26]. **These data suggest that deficiencies in repair of germline DNA damage may contribute to some forms of male factor infertility** (see [4], p. 124).

Another source of DNA error is the recombination process, which involves the events of crossing over and synapsis occurring during meiosis, which evolutionarily allow for DNA variation [3]. Recombination occurs during meiosis prophase I during which a structure termed the synaptonemal complex forms, facilitating the interaction of the maternal and paternal chromosomes. Successful crossover requires a break in the DNA strand necessitating a mechanism to repair that break. This is accomplished via the MLH1 protein, which leaves a detectable mark (foci) on the synaptonemal complex in cases where a successful crossover has occurred. Defects in this process have been linked to examples of male factor infertility suggesting that errors in recombination are linked to male factor infertility in some patients. For example, failure to form a synaptonemal complex was found in a man noted to have meiotic arrest and azoospermia, and associations between reduced recombination frequency and infertility have been reported. Efforts to characterize recombination errors have shown that two types of errors occur – abnormalities in quality and frequency of recombination, both of which happen with more frequency in men with nonobstructive azoospermia [27]. Failure of recombination may also be related to the increased number of aneuploid sperm seen in infertile men. Additional proteins involved in the recombination process have been identified (RAD51, RPA, MSH4, MLH3), which increase the known complexity level of the process. Further research into potential genetic anomalies in these proteins could lead to a better understanding of male factor infertility. The genes involved in this process are still unknown, though one candidate gene is SYCP3 (OMIM 604759, 12q23). Evidence to support a role of the SYCP3 gene in recombination includes observations that male mice cells deficient in this gene do not undergo synapse and meiosis, and a single report of two azoospermic men heterozygous for it.

Anomalies of mitochondrial DNA

Mitochondria are a cell's site of energy production via oxidate phosphorylation using an electron transport chain composed of four complexes (I–IV). Complex V, also located in the mitochondria, is the ATP synthetase. Mitochondria are unique among all cellular organelles as they contain their own genome. This allows them to synthesize proteins without direct control from the nucleus. Interestingly, mitochondrial DNA contains no introns, only exons, meaning that every missense, addition, or deletion has the potential to directly impact the genome's ability to produce the oxidative phosphorylation pathway proteins that are encoded. Additionally, the mitochondrial DNA is attached to the inner membrane of the mitochondrion in close proximity to the respiratory chain and the reactive oxidative species and free radicals produced as by-products. This, along with a relative absence of a basic self-repair mechanism, explains the up to 100-fold increase in mutation rate. Each mammalian sperm contains between 70 and 80 mitochondria in the mid-piece and each of these mitochondria has only one circular piece of DNA. Sperm motility is vital to successful natural fertilization and is dependent on sperm mitochondria to provide adequate energy. Early reports have associated poor sperm motility in 11% and 12% of cases of men with point mutations in the mitochondrion DNA at nucleotides 9055 and 11719, affecting complexes IV and I, respectively [28].

A 2-base-pair deletion affecting nucleotides 8195 and 8196 associated with complex II has also been reported to give rise to a truncated protein and potentially affect sperm motility [29]. A recent study screened 49 men with idiopathic infertility and found that 23 of them had mutations in their mitochondrial DNA [30]. **While mitochondrial DNA mutations may play a significant if not yet fully defined role in cases of idiopathic infertility, such patients would ideally benefit from assisted reproductive techniques, including ICSI, because sperm mitochondria are not passed on to progeny and hence there is no risk of passing on the genetic mutation to the patient's child.**

Conclusions

A complete description of all genetic causes of male factor infertility is not possible in this chapter. With the hard work of numerous researchers, the list of genetic anomalies associated with male infertility increases continuously. Rather, this chapter attempts to highlight some of the more common and better understood genetic anomalies. The interested reader is referred to either [4] or other recently published excellent reviews of the subject for further information [2, 3, 14, 15]. The Online Mendelian Inheritance in Man (OMIM) project (http://www.ncbi.nlm.nih.gov/omim/) is another highly useful resource for the study of genetic defects of all kinds as it provides a searchable, indexed listing of known genetic defects, their etiologies, and their clinical presentation [13].

Modern understanding of the genetic causes of male infertility requires more than simple knowledge of nuclear DNA anomalies and includes variations in mitochondrial DNA, epigenetics, and repair and recombination errors. Basic science continues to advance the understanding of the role that genetics play in the intricate process of reproduction and now includes genes on the X chromosome, which are vital to male fertility. The information in this chapter will assist clinicians as they educate their patients on male fertility and guide their management.

Acknowledgment

Special thanks to Henry M. Rosevear, MD, for his extensive contributions to this chapter.

REFERENCES

[1] Schlegel PN. Evaluation of male infertility. *Minerva Ginecol* 2009; **61**(4): 261–83.

[2] O'Flynn O'Brien KL, Varghese AC, Agarwal A. The genetic causes of male factor infertility: a review. *Fertil Steril* 2010; **93**: 1–12.

[3] Walsh TJ, Pera RR, Turek PJ. The genetics of male infertility. *Semin Reprod Med* 2009; **27**(2): 124–36.

[4] Lipshultz LI, Howards SS, Niederberger CS. *Infertility in the Male*, 4th edn (Cambridge: Cambridge University Press, 2009).

[5] Visootsak J, Graham JM, Jr. Klinefelter syndrome and other sex chromosomal aneuploidies. *Orphanet J Rare Dis* 2006; **1**: 42.

[6] Denschlag D, Tempfer C, Kunze M, Wolff G, Keck C. Assisted reproductive techniques in patients with Klinefelter syndrome: a critical review. *Fertil Steril* 2004; **82**(4): 775–9.

[7] Okada H, Goda K, Yamamoto Y, *et al.* Age as a limiting factor for successful sperm retrieval in patients with nonmosaic Klinefelter's syndrome. *Fertil Steril* 2005; **84**(6): 1662–4.

[8] Ferhi K, Avakian R, Griveau JF, Guille F. Age as only predictive factor for successful sperm recovery in patients with Klinefelter's syndrome. *Andrologia* 2009; **41**(2): 84–7.

[9] Lyon MF. Gene action in the X-chromosome of the mouse (Mus musculus L.). *Nature* 1961; **190**: 372–3.

[10] Martin RH. Cytogenetic determinants of male fertility. *Hum Reprod Update* 2008; **14**(4): 379–90.

[11] Shi Q, Martin RH. Multicolor fluorescence in situ hybridization analysis of meiotic chromosome segregation in a 47,XYY male and a review of the literature. *Am J Med Genet* 2000; **93**: 40–6.

[12] Gantt PA, Byrd JR, Greenblatt RB, McDonough PG. A clinical and cytogenetic study of fifteen patients with 45,X/46XY gonadal dysgenesis. *Fertil Steril* 1980; **34**(3): 216–21.

[13] Hamosh DA. Online Mendelian Inheritance in Man (OMIM) project. 2010.

[14] McLachlan RI, O'Bryan MK. Clinical Review: State of the art for genetic testing of infertile men. *J Clin Endocrinol Metab* 2010; **95**(3): 1013–24.

[15] Poongothai J, Gopenath TS, Manonayaki S. Genetics of human male infertility. *Singapore Med J* 2009; **50**(4): 336–47.

[16] Hopps CV, Mielnik A, Goldstein M, *et al.* Detection of sperm in men with Y chromosome microdeletions of the AZFa, AZFb and AZFc regions. *Hum Reprod* 2003; **18**(8): 1660–5.

[17] Ferlin A, Raicu F, Gatta V, *et al.* Male infertility: role of genetic background. *Reprod Biomed Online* 2007; **14**(6): 734–45.

[18] Vogt PH. Azoospermia factor (AZF) in Yq11: towards a molecular understanding of its function for human male fertility and spermatogenesis. *Reprod Biomed Online* 2005; **10**: 81–93.

[19] Repping S, Skaletsky H, Lange J, *et al.* Recombination between palindromes P5 and P1 on the human Y chromosome causes massive deletions and spermatogenic failure. *Am J Hum Genet* 2002; **71**(4): 906–22.

[20] Oates RD, Silber S, Brown LG, Page DC. Clinical characterization of 42 oligospermic or azoospermic men with microdeletion of the AZFc region of the Y chromosome, and of 18 children conceived via ICSI. *Hum Reprod* 2002; **17**(11): 2813–24.

[21] Lazaros L, Xita N, Kaponis A, *et al.* Evidence for association of sex hormone-binding globulin and androgen receptor genes with semen quality. *Andrologia* 2008; **40**(3): 186–91.

[22] Oakes MB, Eyvazzadeh AD, Quint E, Smith YR. Complete androgen insensitivity syndrome – a review. *J Pediatr Adolesc Gynecol* 2008; **21**(6): 305–10.

[23] Dejager S, Bry-Gauillard H, Bruckert E, *et al.* A comprehensive endocrine description of Kennedy's disease revealing androgen insensitivity linked to CAG repeat length. *J Clin Endocrinol Metab* 2002; **87**(8): 3893–901.

[24] McLachlan RI, Mallidis C, Ma K, Bhasin S, de Kretser DM. Genetic disorders and spermatogenesis. *Reprod Fertil Dev* 1998; **10**: 97–104.

[25] Schlegel PN, Shin D, Goldstein M. Urogenital anomalies in men with congenital absence of the vas deferens. *J Urol* 1996; **155**(5): 1644–8.

[26] Maduro MR, Casella R, Kim E, *et al.* Microsatellite instability and defects in mismatch repair proteins: a new aetiology for Sertoli cell-only syndrome. *Mol Hum Reprod* 2003; **9**(2): 61–8.

[27] Sun F, Greene C, Turek PJ, *et al.* Immunofluorescent synaptonemal complex analysis in azoospermic men. *Cytogenet Genome Res* 2005; **111**(3–4): 366–70.

[28] Holyoake AJ, McHugh P, Wu M, *et al.* High incidence of single nucleotide substitutions in the mitochondrial genome is associated with poor semen parameters in men. *Int J Androl* 2001; **24**(3): 175–82.

[29] Thangaraj K, Joshi MB, Reddy AG, *et al.* Sperm mitochondrial mutations as a cause of low sperm motility. *J Androl* 2003; **24**(3): 388–92.

[30] Kumar R, Bhat A, Bamezai RN, *et al.* Necessity of nuclear and mitochondrial genome analysis prior to assisted reproductive techniques/intracytoplasmic sperm injection. *Indian J Biochem Biophys* 2007; **44**(6): 437–42.

(a)

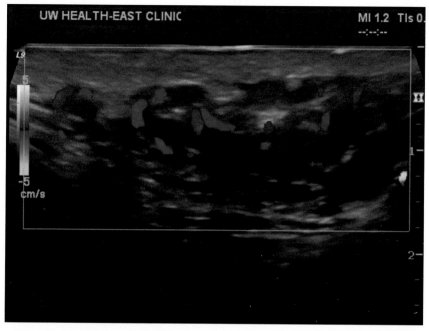

(b)

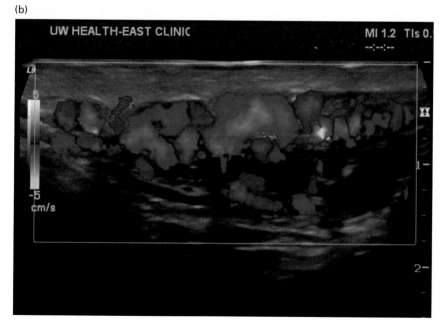

Figure 3.1 Duplex ultrasound of varicocele (a) at rest and (b) with Valsalva maneuver.

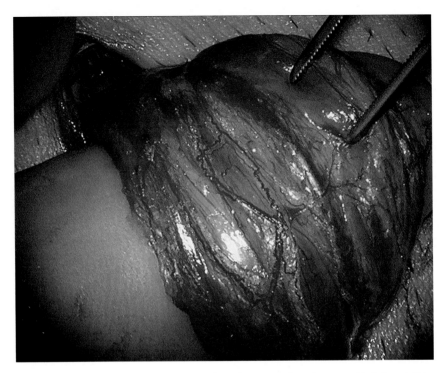

Figure 3.2 Spermatic cord structures as seen through an operating microscope (8×). From left to right: lymphatic (shiny, clear), vas deferens (white), vein (blue), testicular artery (dark red), vein (blue, under tips of forceps), vein (blue, behind forceps).

(a)

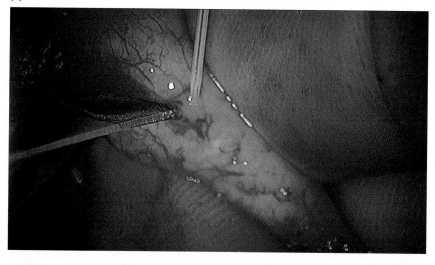

(b)

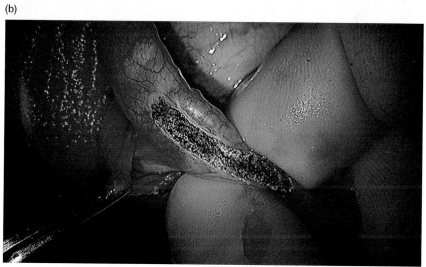

Figure 3.3 Microsurgical epididymal sperm aspiration (MESA). (a) An ophthalmological blade is used to open the delicate epididymal tubules while fluid is aspirated into an angiocath-tipped syringe. (b) Appearance of epididymis upon completion of an "obliterative" MESA.

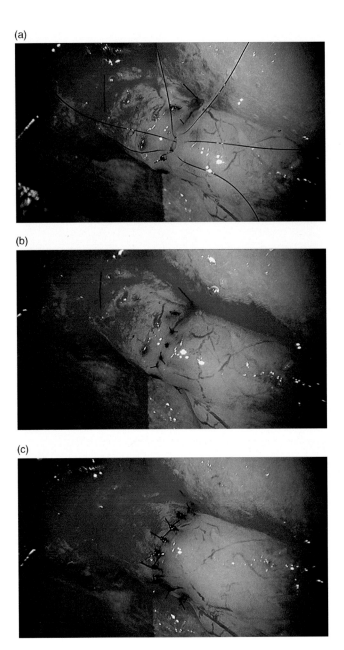

Figure 3.5 Microsurgical, two-layer vasovasostomy. (a) The posterior outer seromuscular and inner mucosal layers have been tied. The inner mucosal layer sutures of 10-0 nylon are individually placed anteriorly giving a "spider's web" appearance. (b) Inner mucosal sutures tied. (c) Outer seromuscular sutures of 9-0 nylon tied to create a watertight closure.

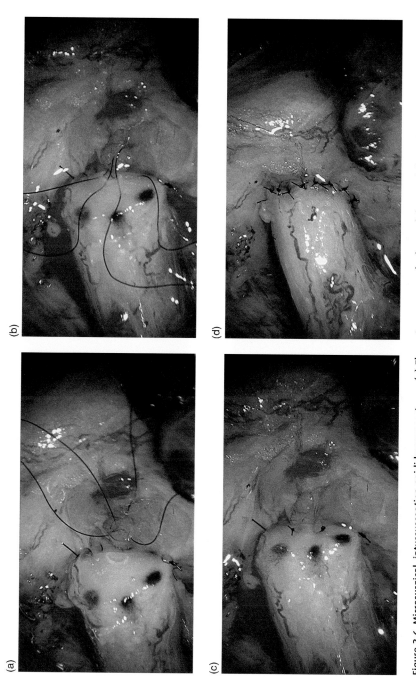

Figure 3.6 Microsurgical, intussusception epididymovasostomy. (a) The outer seromuscular layer of the vas deferens has been secured to the tunica of the epididymis with 9-0 nylon sutures. Double-armed 10-0 nylon sutures have been placed in an epididymal tubule. The tubule has been opened, and the presence of sperm has been confirmed. (b) The 10-0 nylon sutures are placed in the lumen of the vas deferens. (c) 10-0 nylon sutures tied, thereby intussuscepting the opened epididymal tubule into the lumen of the vas deferens. (d) The outer seromuscular layer of the vas deferens is anastamosed to the epididymal tunica with interrupted 9-0 nylon sutures.

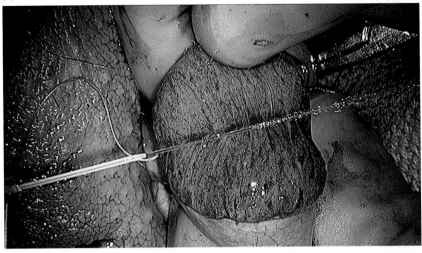

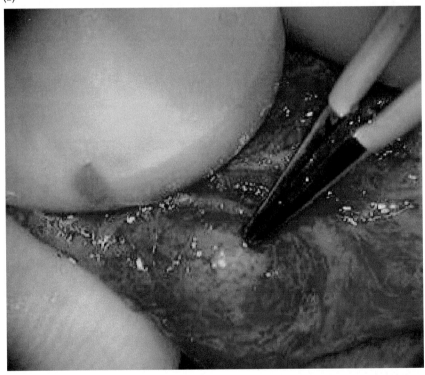

Figure 3.7 Microdissection testicular sperm extraction (micro-TESE). (a) The tunica albuginea is opened along the equator of the testicle under low power. (b) Under higher-power optical magnification, seminiferous tubules that are believed to have active spermatogenesis (at tips of bipolar forceps) are seen as being "full" relative to the smaller "empty" tubules around them.

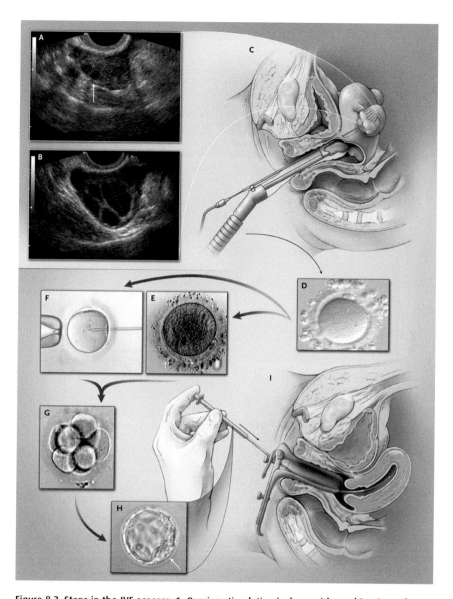

Figure 8.3 Steps in the IVF process: 1. Ovarian stimulation is done with combinations of injectable drugs for several weeks. The goal is to get many follicles developing so that eggs can be retrieved. In the figure above, A shows an ultrasound view of an unstimulated ovary. B is the same ovary after several days of stimulation. The black ovals are fluid-filled ovarian follicles that contain eggs. 2. Once the eggs are thought to be mature based on ultrasound measurements of the follicles, egg retrieval is performed under ultrasound guidance (C). This step is performed with sedatives and pain medications. 3. The retrieved eggs (D) are next fertilized in the laboratory, either by mixing eggs with sperm in a culture dish (E) or by injecting a single sperm into the egg (F) by a process called intracytoplasmic injection. 4. The resulting embryos are then cultured for several days (G is a 3-day-old eight-cell embryo, H is a 5-day-old blastocyst embryo) before the best embryos are selected to be transferred back to the uterus(I).

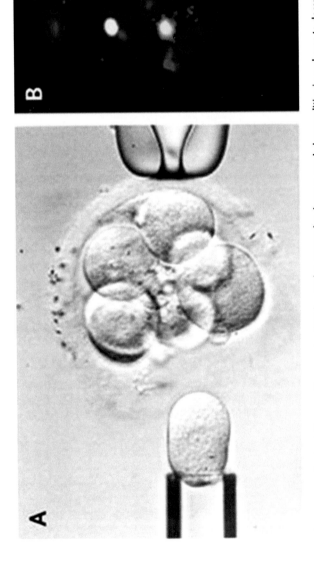
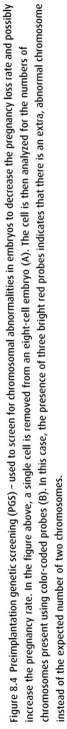

Figure 8.4 Preimplantation genetic screening (PGS) – used to screen for chromosomal abnormalities in embryos to decrease the pregnancy loss rate and possibly increase the pregnancy rate. In the figure above, a single cell is removed from an eight-cell embryo (A). The cell is then analyzed for the numbers of chromosomes present using color-coded probes (B). In this case, the presence of three bright red probes indicates that there is an extra, abnormal chromosome instead of the expected number of two chromosomes.

7

Semen: analysis and processing

Grace M. Centola, PhD, HCLD (ABB)

Semen analysis is often the first test ordered when a couple presents for infertility evaluation. **Along with evaluation of the female partner (see Chapter 8 in this book), semen analysis can provide valuable information to the physician who can then formulate a treatment plan.** Semen analysis, however, can only provide information on the *potential* for fertility (i.e., normal-appearing, motile sperm are present and the testes are producing sperm). Semen analysis alone cannot demonstrate that sperm are able to successfully fertilize a mature oocyte given the appropriate environment. More detailed functional testing (see below) may be warranted, based on overall medical, social, and sexual history, and other testing of the couple.

Semen quality has been called a "surrogate measure" of male fertility potential, a marker of injury, toxic exposures (drugs, endocrine disrupters, heavy metals), infections, fever, and even psychosocial stress [1]. **Semen analysis provides information on health of the testes, adequacy of the endocrine system, and health of the accessory organs producing the fluid bathing sperm in the ejaculate** [1]. Semen analysis provides information on sperm production by the testes, spermiogenesis, or sperm maturation as evidenced by sperm morphology, sperm function demonstrated by motility (and thus potential ability to swim through the female reproductive tract towards the oocyte), and lastly, secretion of the genital tract accessory glands. First and foremost, semen analysis can tell the physician that the testes are producing motile sperm in sufficient numbers to reach a threshold that spills into ejaculatory fluid. Semen analysis can not, however, tell which of those sperm can actually make it to the egg, penetrate egg vestments, and initiate the subsequent fertilization processes.

In order for the results of semen analysis to be clinically valid, testing should be done in a clinical laboratory, with specific instructions given to the

An Introduction to Male Reproductive Medicine, ed. Craig Niederberger. Published by Cambridge University Press. © Cambridge University Press 2011.

patient regarding abstinence, specimen collection, and specimen transport.
Sure, anyone can put a smear of semen onto a slide and determine that motile
sperm are present, but are they present in enough numbers and quality with the
potential for fertilization? At home, semen analysis kits are available that change
color if sperm are present at a threshold number causing the color change, much
like a pregnancy test. This information may certainly be a starting point, but
additional basic information will be needed, including percentage of moving
sperm, percentage of morphologically normal sperm, presence of round cells and
possibly bacteria, semen volume, color, and pH, all of which are part of a
standard semen analysis.

**Although numbers are important, it is the quality of individual sperm, and
their functional ability that is ultimately the determining factor for male
fertility potential. Semen characteristics can be widely variable [4], and there
is overlap between fertile and infertile men [4].** It is recommended to have at
least three semen analyses, with 2–3 weeks minimum between each test. Others
recommend at least two analyses and a third if the first two are significantly
different [4]. One recent study showed that in at least 85% of cases, one analysis
(of the first semen sample) is predictive of subsequent semen analyses [7].
Interpretation of the test results completes the analysis and provides a basis
upon which the physician can provide advice and direction to the couple. While
semen analysis provides useful information to the clinician, the combination of
several parameters is more predictive of a couple's fertility potential [6, 8].
Semen analysis has been referred to as an important piece in the jigsaw puzzle
for the clinician to evaluate along with patient history, physical, and hormone
analyses (see Chapters 2 and 8 in this book and [9], chapter 10).

Semen analysis

Abstinence and collection

**In order for semen analysis to provide useful and reliable clinical informa-
tion, it is extremely important that the semen sample be collected properly,
that methods for analysis are accurate, and results are properly interpreted.**
The importance of specific instructions to the patient regarding abstinence
period, specimen collection, and transport cannot be overemphasized. There
should be a standardized abstinence period of 2–5 days from the previous
ejaculation (see [9], chapter 33, p. 551); the WHO manual recommends a
minimum of 2 days with a maximum of 7 days [4]. The old wives tale that
longer abstinence allows one to "save it all up" is misleading and incorrect! The
longer the abstinence period, the ejaculate becomes filled with dead and dying
sperm as well as non-motile sperm (reduced overall percentage motility), and
thus, not a true picture of semen quality [10] (see also [9], p. 551).

**A comfortable and professional collection room should be provided for
specimen collection (see [9], chapter 33, p. 551).** An accessible washroom,

seating as well as magazines and videos are helpful for comfort and stimulation, which allows optimum specimen collection. Collection at the laboratory facility allows control of the time to analysis and proper holding temperature before analysis [4]. The specimen should be collected by masturbation without the use of lubricants. However, some men are unable to collect by masturbation and, therefore, a non-toxic condom can be provided for use with sexual intercourse. There is some evidence that semen samples collected at home were of better quality than those collected at the clinic, and this may be due to a less stressful environment [11]. If collected at home, the specimen should be kept warm, close to body temperature, and delivered to the laboratory within 1 h of collection.

Laboratory analysis

Upon receipt of the specimen by the laboratory, a period of at least 30 min from ejaculation time is needed for semen to liquefy from a coagulated state, to a more liquid state, which is easier to manipulate for analysis. Semen is examined by drawing into a pipette, to determine if liquefaction is complete or partial or even delayed over time, as well as the consistency or viscosity of semen. Viscosity is the homogeneous thickness of semen, and does not change with time [4]. Decreased motility can be a result of partial or non-liquefaction, or increased viscosity (see [9], chapter 33).

Macroscopic examination of semen color is important. Yellow or green-tinged semen may be indicative of infection, brown-colored semen is often seen in spinal cord injured men (see [9], chapter 33), and reddish-tinged semen may result from the presence of red blood cells. **Normal semen color is opaque and gray–white in color.** Clear semen can be indicative of a severely low sperm count, or azoospermia [13].

Measurement of semen pH is no longer routinely recommended, particularly if sperm are present (see [9], p. 552). Semen pH can vary with time from ejaculation, exposure to ambient air or differences in holding temperature and thus can be highly inaccurate. **In the case of low semen volume or azoospermia, for example, measurement of seminal pH can be indicative of accessory gland dysfunction or duct obstruction, but other biochemical tests or physical examination may be more reliable (see [9], chapter 33) and informative.**

Initial analysis involves scanning an entire wet-mount slide of a drop of semen to examine for presence of sperm, but also presence of excessive debris, bacteria, and round cells. Excessive round cells, which may be white blood cells (WBCs) or immature sperm should be confirmed by special staining, which is available in specialized clinical andrology laboratories (see [9], chapter 38). Peroxidase staining can be used to detect granulocytes, but will not account for other leukocytes such as monocytes, which can account for half of the total WBC count [4] (see also [9], chapter 38). The normal concentration for WBCs in semen has been arbitrarily set at 1 million per milliliter [4, 5]. Although the peroxidase stain is the method of choice for WBC determination in semen, other stains, including special immunocytochemical stains and flow cytometry, have shown some promise for determining WBCs in semen (see also [9], chapter 38). The presence of increased numbers of WBCs is not always associated with infection. However, increased leukocytes on repeated examinations should be further checked, as they are associated with poor semen quality because of increased oxygen radicals or reactive oxygen species (see also [9], chapter 39).

Examination of sperm count and motility is most often performed using specialized counting chambers such as a hemocytometer or Makler counting chamber. **The numbers of moving sperm as well as non-moving sperm are counted, and based on dilution factors, the total sperm concentration in millions per milliliter and the percentage of moving sperm (motility) can be calculated.** With the semen volume, the total sperm count is calculated as well as a total motile count.

Computer-assisted semen analysis has been used in some laboratories for routine analysis and is thought by many to be reliable and reproducible. **With automated systems, a specialized computer is used to track motile sperm and provide sperm count, motility, speed, and quality of sperm movement** [4]. However, these automated analyzers are quite expensive as well as difficult to set-up, use, and standardize in the busy clinical laboratory. Thus the potential of computer-assisted semen analysis has not been realized, and has not provided significant advantage over current manual assessment of sperm count and motility (see [9], chapter 33).

Sperm morphology

An important part of routine semen analysis is the determination of the numbers of normal-appearing sperm using a specially stained slide preparation. It is not possible to obtain a reliable sperm morphology on an unstained wet-mount preparation or prestained slides. While some consider sperm morphology to be able to predict fertilization rate and pregnancy outcome in assisted reproduction, others question its relevance [13]. (See also [9], chapter 34.) Standardized and reliable methods for determining sperm morphology should be used to assess sperm shape. Classification of sperm morphology has developed significantly over the years, from the earlier traditional methods of MacLeod [15] and Eliasson [1], to guidelines from the World Health Organization [4] and strict criteria for morphology assessment [14, 16]. (See also [9], chapter 34.) (Comparison of the strict criteria and WHO classification methods of morphology are demonstrated in [9], table 34.1, chapter 34.) The most recent edition of the WHO semen analysis manual utilizes a morphology classification that is more closely related to the strict criteria of assessment [4]. These methodologies classify "normal" spermatozoa as those demonstrating a specific head size and shape, a straight, regular mid-piece, and slender, uncoiled tail. Under strict criteria, sperm is normal if its conformation agrees exactly with four strict criteria; those not conforming to these criteria are classified as abnormal.

WHO criteria for assessing male fertility potential

Normal ranges

The *WHO Manual for the Laboratory Examination of Human Semen and Sperm–Cervical Mucus Interaction* ("The WHO Manual") was initially published in 1980, and has undergone revisions in 1992, 1999, and, most recently, 2010 [4]. **This manual has become a globally accepted reference manual for semen analysis, sperm function testing, and andrology laboratory procedures, and has set the standard for what is considered to be the "normal fertile range," or rather, parameters below which, a man would be considered "infertile."** Previous versions of this manual, although widely used, have had serious limitations as data were derived from non-standardized populations and from laboratories that were not well controlled [2]. Cooper *et al.* examined semen parameters from over 4500 men in 14 countries and conducted exhaustive statistical analyses with 95% confidence limits to provide sound reference distributions of semen characteristics, which have become the basis for the most recent, year 2010 edition of the WHO manual [2].

Table 7.1 summarizes the normal ranges as reported in the most recent version of the WHO manual. It is important to consider that these values are only a guide to a man's fertility status and if values fall within the 95% confidence limits, fertility is not guaranteed. To be clinically valid, the results of two or more semen analyses must be digested in context with the entire clinical picture of both the male and female partner. **Given that the analysis reports on anywhere from 3 to 10 or more sperm parameters, there are multiple combinations of so-called defects that may contribute to a man's subfertility or fertility potential.** Table 7.2 lists the more important terms routinely used to characterize a man's semen analysis or clinical impression. It is important to note that the term "zoospermia" refers to the spermatozoa, and "spermia" refers more generally to the ejaculate. The most common recognizable term, azoospermia, refers to the absence of spermatozoa in the ejaculate, but "cryptozoospermia" refers to the presence of sperm in a centrifuged specimen, but not on a standard wet-mount examination.

Men whose semen parameters fall below the threshold value for "normal range" are not necessarily infertile, but fall out of the range of men who were recently fertile and who participated in the population studies that contributed to the WHO ranges. **Those who fall out of the normal range may be helped by medical therapies (see Chapter 4 in this book), or more or less invasive assisted reproductive technologies (ARTs) based on the overall couple's clinical picture.**

A clinician reviewing and interpreting the results of a patient's semen analysis should also consider possible regional and seasonal differences in sperm parameters, as well as possible differences in laboratory expertise [4]. **Many laboratories establish specific "in-house" normal ranges that will account for regional and inherent laboratory variations, which will then assist the physician with directing the couple to the most likely means to achieve their goal of a pregnancy.**

Table 7.1 WHO Normal Ranges. Data from reference [4]

	Parameter	5th centile range
Semen volume	1.5 ml	1.4–1.7
Sperm count no./ejaculate	39×10^6	33–46
Sperm concentration no./ml	15×10^6	12–16
Progressive motility (%)	32%	31–34
Total motility (progressive + non-progressive motile)	40%	38–42
Viability (vitality) % live	58%	55–63
Normal morphology (%)	4%	3.0–4.0
	Other threshold values from the WHO consensus	
pH	≥ 7.2	
White blood cell concentration	$<1 \times 10^6$	
% Antibody positive by mixed antiglobulin reaction screen or immunobead test screen	$<50\%$	
Seminal zinc	≥ 2.4	
Fructose concentration	≥ 13 μmol/ejaculate	
Neutral glucosidase	≥ 20 mU/ejaculate	

Table 7.2 Common terminology. Data from reference [4]

Term	Definition
Aspermia	No semen or ejaculate produced. There may be retrograde ejaculation (into the bladder)
Normozoospermia	Normal sperm count, motility, and morphology
Oligozoospermia	Decreased total number of sperm
Asthenozoospermia	Decreased percentage motility
Teratozoospermia	Decreased percentage normal forms
Asthenoteratozoospermia	Decreased percentage motility and normal forms
Oligoasthenozoospermia	Decreased number of sperm and decreased percentage motility
Oligoasthenoteratozoospermia	Decreased number of sperm, percentage motility, and percentage normal forms
Azoospermia	No sperm in the ejaculate
Cryptozoospermia	No sperm seen in the ejaculate, but sperm found in a centrifuged pellet
Hematospermia	Presence of red blood cells in semen
Leukocytospermia, pyospermia	Presence of white blood cells in semen
Necrozoospermia	Decreased percentage live sperm and increased percentage immotile sperm

The results of semen analyses, in conjunction with physical examination, other tests, and tests on the woman, need to be interpreted logically and intelligently. For example, in a man with a low sperm count and low motility, with a completely normal female partner, a physician might consider intrauterine insemination (IUI). In cases where there is a low sperm count, low motility, and low percentage of normal forms, and a normal woman, or even a woman with ovulatory dysfunction, the couple may be treated both medically and with IUI, or even in vitro fertilization (IVF). In cases of azoospermia, medical and/or surgical treatment may be acceptable, but if not, use of donor sperm insemination may be the only possibility for the couple to experience a pregnancy. The reader is directed to sperm processing (below) as well as Chapters 2, 3, and 4 in this book, and in [9] (chapters 21, 22, 35, and 36) for comprehensive reviews of medical and surgical options based on testing results of both partners.

Other tests of male fertility potential

In the absence of an obvious defect on a semen analysis test, it is often advantageous to conduct more advanced testing that would give additional detail for the clinician to utilize in formulating a treatment paradigm. A common test in the andrology laboratory is a test for the presence of antisperm antibodies [4] (see also [9], chapter 37). Antisperm antibodies are of the immunoglobulin class type IgG and IgA, and these can be present on the spermatozoa (head, tail, mid-piece), as well as in the seminal fluid, cervical mucus, and follicular fluid and serum. **Antisperm antibodies can cause sperm clumping or agglutination and decreased motility, as well as interfere with sperm–egg binding, and even with post-fertilization events, including embryo cleavage and development.** However, such defects in sperm function are not exclusively a result of the presence of antisperm antibodies. Thus, interpretation of antibody testing must be taken with caution, and within the context of standard semen analysis and possibly other more advanced tests of sperm function. Direct and indirect tests for the presence of antisperm antibodies are commercially available and relatively easy to perform [4].

Additional testing would center on tests of important sperm function such as sperm–zona pellucida binding, sperm penetration assay, capacitation assays, and acrosome reaction assays [17]. Cellular or fertility markers also include chemical induction of the sperm acrosome reaction, hypo-osmotic swelling of the sperm cell membrane, and assessment of sperm DNA damage. Levels of these markers may have a direct or indirect relationship to necessary sperm functions, and the absence of such markers or characteristics would preclude normal fertilization [17].

Additionally, measurement of oxygen radicals – reactive oxygen species (ROS) – has emerged as important ancillary testing as these free radicals may play a role in spermatozoa damage and in seminal oxidative stress (see [9], chapter 39). Immature sperm and leukocytes appear to be the main source of ROS.

Levels of these markers may have a direct or indirect relationship to necessary sperm functions, and the absence of such markers or characteristics would preclude normal fertilization. Admittedly, however, measurement of oxidative stress and ROS levels are beyond the scope of the conventional sperm function tests and general andrology laboratory (see [9], chapter 39).

With the advent of assisted reproduction, particularly intracytoplasmic sperm injection (ICSI), abnormal sperm function could be bypassed, with the sperm placed directly into the egg, thereby negating all of the steps necessary before penetration of the oocyte. The use of advanced sperm function testing has decreased significantly since the routine use of ICSI [17]. However, unexpected failure of fertilization following ICSI, particularly in the so-called normal man, and failure of pregnancy following transfer of good-quality embryos, leaves many unanswered questions. Sperm with normal morphology are not always able to function properly, even once placed into the cytoplasm of the oocyte. **More advanced sperm function tests may be able to shed light on the reason behind many sperm function defects.**

Table 7.3 lists several of the more common sperm function tests. These tests include assessment of sperm DNA damage, membrane function (swelling in hypo-osmotic buffer), cervical mucus penetration, sperm binding to the zona pellucida, sperm penetration into zona-free hamster oocytes, special staining for the sperm acrosome, and induction of sperm capacitation and acrosome reaction [17] (see also [9], chapter 40). Unfortunately, **the current clinical utility of many of these advanced tests is limited and available only in select specialized laboratories. Most of these tests become clinically relevant in cases of unexplained infertility that may be attributed to the sperm, particularly in cases of unexpected fertilization failure in IVF/ICSI.**

Sperm processing: intrauterine insemination and assisted reproductive technologies

Artificial insemination, specifically, cervical insemination, has been a routine practice since the late 1800s or even earlier. The use of IUI, which places motile sperm directly through the cervix into the uterine cavity, has been widely utilized since the mid-1980s with the introduction of ARTs. IUI is useful in many cases of subfertility, but especially in cases of sperm–cervical mucus hostility, decreased sperm motility, and decreased sperm concentration. **IUI allows a concentrated fraction of motile spermatozoa to be deposited directly into the uterus, giving the sperm "a head start."** If the insemination is performed at the appropriate mid-cycle time, adequate pregnancy success has been reported, even with severely oligozoospermic men.

In order to place the sperm directly into the uterine cavity, the function of the female cervix must be mimicked, and this is accomplished by "sperm washing" or sperm processing. The fresh ejaculate contains many contaminants, such as dead and dying sperm, cellular debris, bacteria, epithelial cells, and WBCs, and

Table 7.3 Common sperm function tests. Data from reference [4]

Sperm function test	What the test measures
Peroxidase stain	Polymorphonuclear neutrophils/ neutrophils in semen
CD45 monoclonal antibody staining	Distinguishes between leukocytes and germ cells in the semen
Hypo-osmotic swelling test (HOS Test)	Ability of the sperm to swell in a hypo-osmotic buffer is directly related to proper function of the sperm plasma membrane, and related to ability of the sperm to complete the capacitation process and successfully penetrate an oocyte
Antisperm antibody Mixed antiglobulin reaction screen	Direct test for presence of IgG and IgA on the surface of sperm in freshly ejaculated semen
Antisperm antibody IBT	Direct test for presence of IgG and IgA on the surface of washed sperm. The IBT can also be used as an "indirect" test to determine the presence of antibodies in sperm-free fluid (e.g., serum, cervical mucus, follicular fluid)

Sperm–cervical mucus interaction tests
  Postcoital test – in vivo test
  Simple slide test
  Kremer capillary tube test
  Penetrak test kit
	Ability of sperm to penetrate the mid-cycle cervical mucus. In vivo test – sample of cervical mucus taken following coitus. In vitro tests – ability of sperm to penetrate test or donor cervical mucus on a slide or in a capillary tube

Seminal zinc	Function of the prostate gland that contributes zinc to the seminal fluid
Seminal fructose	Presence of, and proper function of the seminal vesicles that contribute fructose to the seminal fluid
L-carnitine/glycerophosphocholine, neutral α-glucosidase	Presence in seminal fluid as a function of the epididymis
Sperm motion parameters – computer-assisted semen analysis	Sperm motion kinetics, such as velocity or speed, straightness of sperm track, movement of the sperm head during swimming

Reactive oxygen species
  Chemiluminescence
  Nitroblue tetrazolium staining
  Cytochrome *c* reduction test
  Flow cytometry
	Presence of oxygen radicals in the semen, contributed by dead/dying sperm cells and leukocytes. Hinders function of normal spermatozoa; membrane damage, nuclear and mitochondrial DNA damage

Hemi-zona assay	Ability of sperm to bind to the oocyte zona pellucida

Table 7.3 (*cont.*)

Sperm function test	What the test measures
Zona-free hamster penetration assay (sperm penetration assay)	Ability of sperm to penetrate zona pellucida-free hamster eggs and decondense in the egg cytoplasm
Acrosome status and induced acrosome reaction	Ability of the sperm to complete the process of capacitation and shed the acrosomal cap
DNA status/DNA damage	Special staining and use of flow cytometry to determine the presence of damaged DNA. Methods include Sperm Chromatin Structure Assay (SCSA^{TM}), and the TUNEL assay

IBT, immunobead binding test.

prostaglandins. Normally, these seminal components do not pass through the cervix. **Washing procedures mimic the function of the female cervix.**

Therefore, in order to perform an IUI, sperm must be removed from the seminal fluid and placed into a nutrient medium that is conducive to sperm survival, and may in fact stimulate sperm motility and function. The motile sperm are concentrated into a small volume of nutrient medium, which can be easily placed into the uterine cavity with little or no discomfort to the female patient. The washing procedure resuspends the spermatozoa in medium that contains nutrients, which can stimulate sperm function and motility, and enhance sperm longevity in the female reproductive tract. Additives to the nutrient medium have been shown to benefit poor specimens and improve sperm fertilizability. Likewise, in order to use the spermatozoa for IVF and ICSI, they must be washed free of seminal fluid contaminants, and suspended in the nutrient medium. An appropriate concentration of washed motile sperm can be mixed with the oocytes in a laboratory dish, or a selected normal sperm in the case of ICSI can then be picked up into a special pipette and injected into the oocyte.

There are many different laboratory procedures used to process or "wash" sperm for IUI and IVF/ICSI. Methods include simple washing–centrifugation, swim-up from a (centrifuged) pellet of sperm or swim-up from the semen itself in a test-tube, and density gradient centrifugation [4]. **Density gradient centrifugation is the most common sperm processing procedure, especially in specimens demonstrating normal sperm concentration but high levels of cellular contaminants and debris.** The simple washing–centrifugation procedure is best utilized for semen specimens of higher quality with little contamination, and is useful when the sperm concentration is low. A swim-up procedure, based on the ability of motile sperm to swim out of the seminal fluid, is also useful in specimens with higher levels of contaminating cells and debris. These techniques for sperm processing are routinely utilized for IUI and IVF.

The method of choice is determined by sperm motility, concentration, and quality, as well as the subsequent use of the processed sperm. For use with IVF/ICSI, a density gradient wash is most often followed by a swim-up as this will yield a very clean, highly motile sperm population (with little or no contamination with cell debris, or gradient components that can be toxic to oocytes and embryos) [4, 18]. Use of a density gradient also avoids centrifugation of the heterogeneous seminal fluid (i.e., containing motile and non-motile sperm, debris, bacteria, round cells, and WBCs). Centrifuging such a population of live and dead or dying cells increases the production of ROS, which is harmful to live motile sperm. For a detailed description of sperm processing procedures, the reader is also directed to [9] (chapter 35).

Cryopreservation of ejaculated and testicular sperm

Semen cryopreservation is a relatively routine procedure available in most specialized andrology and ART laboratories [4]. (See also [9], chapter 36.). With the advent of assisted reproduction, most particularly ICSI, small numbers of sperm are needed, and thus, cryopreservation of most any ejaculate, testicular tissue, and epididymal aspirates may yield enough sperm to attempt these ART procedures [19].

Semen cryopreservation is also routinely used before: chemotherapy and radiation for cancer treatment; military deployment; chemical or pesticide exposures; and surgical treatments such as vasectomy [4, 19]. Cryopreservation and 180-day quarantine of donor semen has been the industry standard practice mandated by state regulations since the late 1980s, and more recently (2005) by federal regulations. A man may also elect to freeze and store semen to store multiple specimens in an attempt to increase sperm concentration for insemination as well as in times of his physical absence at the time of ovulation or ART procedure [4].

Semen is cryopreserved in liquid nitrogen (liquid or vapor phase) using a cryoprotectant chemical such as glycerol to protect the cells from damage due to intracellular ice crystal formation. The semen is mixed with the cryopreservative, loaded into special cryovials or straws, and then submerged into the liquid nitrogen. The sperm are held in this state of suspended animation, and have been known to thaw with maintenance of fertilizing function for more than 15 years. Following thaw, the semen can be artificially inseminated, or "washed" and prepared for IUI or IVF/ICSI.

If raw semen is frozen, a washing procedure must be employed upon semen thaw in order to use the sperm for IUI or IVF/ICSI. Spermatozoa can also be washed free of the seminal fluid, then frozen as "IUI-ready" vials. These specimens can be thawed and inseminated (IUI) without further processing.

Surgically retrieved spermatozoa (microscopic epididymal sperm aspiration specimens), or testicular biopsy tissue can also be successfully cryopreserved and thawed for use in IVF/ICSI (see Chapter 3 in this book, and chapter 26 in [9]).

Surgical retrieval can be done in cases of obstructive and non-obstructive azoospermia, and can yield enough numbers of sperm for IVF/ICSI. **Cryopreservation of testicular biopsy specimens and epididymal aspirates retrieved at the time of surgical exploration for diagnosis and possible correction of obstruction is advantageous in that sperm can be stored frozen alleviating the need for future surgeries if the obstruction is not corrected.** Multiple vials of retrieved spermatozoa can usually be stored, which allows multiple attempts at IVF/ICSI procedures. Furthermore, cryopreservation at the time of surgical intervention negates the need for synchronous treatment of the female partner, and insures the presence of the partner's sperm at the time of the woman's ovarian stimulation and egg retrieval [9], pages 593–600.

Summary and conclusions

Routine semen analysis provides a wealth of information if interpreted correctly and utilized appropriately to manage the infertile man. Semen analysis gives information on sperm production by the testes, maturation, and acquisition of capacity to swim, but does not give information on the functional ability of the spermatozoa to penetrate an oocyte and perform functions once in oocyte cytoplasm. More advanced sperm function tests can be used by the clinician to gain information on the ability of spermatozoa to complete selected processes necessary to bind to the egg, penetrate egg vestments, and join with the egg nucleus.

Over the last 20 or more years, techniques for washing spermatozoa from seminal fluid, concentrating numbers of motile sperm and stimulating sperm function have been developed, which allow for insemination of sperm directly into the uterine cavity, as well as for use in assisted reproduction. **Such procedures have been used to assist couples presenting with suboptimal sperm concentration and/or motility. Sperm washing allows the use of even a severely impaired semen sample for the treatment of male subfertility.**

Semen cryopreservation, employed for over 50 years, is mandated for anonymous donor semen use, and has been routinely used to maintain fertility potential (e.g., "fertility insurance"), following medical and surgical treatments that may reduce or affect a man's fertility. Sperm banking is also an effective tool in the clinicians' armamentarium for the treatment of male factor infertility.

REFERENCES

[1] Eliasson R. Semen analysis with regard to sperm number, sperm morphology and functional aspects. *Asian J Androl* 2010; **12**: 26–32.

[2] Cooper T, Noonan E, von Eckardstein S, *et al.* World Health Organization reference values for human semen characteristics. *Hum Reprod Update* 2010; **16**(3): 231–45.

[3] Gollenberg AL, Liu F, Brazil C, *et al.* Semen quality in fertile men in relation to psychosocial stress. *Fertil Steril* 2010; **93**(4): 1104–11.

[4] World Health Organization. *WHO Manual for the Examination and Processing of Human Semen*, 5th edn (Geneva: WHO Press, 2010).

[5] Bjorndahl L. Semen analysis: essentials for the clinician. In *Reproductive Endocrinology and Infertility: Integrating Modern Clinical and Laboratory Practice*, Carrell DT, Peterson CM, eds (New York: Springer, 2010), pp. 379–88.

[6] Poch MA, Sigman M. Clinical evaluation and treatment of male factor infertility. In *Reproductive Endocrinology and Infertility: Integrating Modern Clinical and Laboratory Practice*, Carrell DT, Peterson CM, eds (New York: Springer, 2010), pp. 367–78.

[7] Rylander L, Wetterstrand B, Haugen TB, *et al.* Single semen analysis as a predictor of semen quality: clinical and epidemiological implications. *Asian J Androl* 2009; **11**(6): 723–30.

[8] Guzick DS, Overstreet JW, Factor-Litvak P, *et al.* Sperm morphology, motility and concentration in fertile and infertile men. *N Engl J Med* 2001; **345**(19): 1388–93.

[9] Lipshultz L, Howards S, Niederberger C. *Infertility in the Male*, 4th edn (Cambridge: Cambridge University Press, 2009).

[10] Levitas E, Lunenfeld E, Weiss N, *et al.* Relationship between the duration of sexual abstinence and semen quality: analysis of 9,489 semen samples. *Fertil Steril* 2005; **83**: 1680–6.

[11] Elzanaty S, Malm J. Comparison of semen parameters in samples collected by masturbation at a clinic and at home. *Fertil Steril* 2008; **89**(6): 1718–22.

[12] Shetty Licht R, Handle L, Sigman M. Site of semen collection and its effect on semen analysis parameters. *Fertil Steril* 2008; **89**(2): 395–7.

[13] Centola GM. Routine semen analysis. In *Evaluation and Treatment of the Infertile Male*, Centola GM, Ginsburg KA, eds (Cambridge: Cambridge University Press, 1996), pp. 19–29.

[14] Kruger TF, Menkveld R, Stander F, *et al.* Sperm morphologic features as a prognostic factor in in vitro fertilization. *Fertil Steril* 1986; **46**: 1118–23.

[15] MacLeod J. A testicular response during and following a severe allergic reaction. *Fertil Steril* 1962; **13**: 531–41.

[16] Kruger TF, Acosta AA, Simmons KF *et al.* Predictive value of abnormal sperm morphology in in vitro fertilization. *Fertil Steril* 1988; **49**: 112–17.

[17] Alukal JP, Lamb DJ. Advanced tests of sperm function. In *Reproductive Endocrinology and Infertility: Integrating Modern Clinical and Laboratory Practice*, Carrell DT, Peterson CM, eds (New York: Springer, 2010), pp. 423–9.

[18] Centola GM. Sperm preparation for insemination. In *Office Andrology*, Patton PE, Battaglia DE, eds (Totowa: Humana Press, 2005), pp. 39–52.

[19] Centola GM. Sperm banking, donation and transport in the age of assisted reproduction: Federal and State Regulation. In *Reproductive Endocrinology and Infertility: Integrating Modern Clinical and Laboratory Practice*, Carrell DT, Peterson CM, eds (New York: Springer, 2010), pp. 509–16.

8

What to know about the infertile female

Bradley J. Van Voorhis, MD

The physician evaluating the male partner of an infertile couple must know about the female partner's medical and reproductive history. Before any major intervention for infertility (e.g., varicocele repair) is contemplated in the man, the urologist must know whether or not the female partner is, in fact, capable of conceiving a pregnancy following the procedure. **Ideally, there should be a close working relationship between the urologist and gynecologist when taking care of the infertile couple.** In this chapter, I hope to succinctly summarize the important aspects of female fertility and infertility.

As a reproductive endocrinologist, I approach the infertile couple by testing each of three areas that can have major effects on fertility for a couple: sperm production, ovulation, and female pelvic anatomy, including patency of the fallopian tubes. Severe abnormalities in any of these areas can lead to sterility with no hope of achieving a pregnancy without the aid of assisted reproductive techniques. Often more subtle defects are present in one or more of these areas, which contribute to a condition of subfertility, meaning that a natural pregnancy may take significantly longer to achieve. Besides these "big 3" factors, female age is a fourth factor that affects all our infertility evaluation and treatment strategies. Societal shifts towards later marriage and delayed childbearing has led to increasing pressure to achieve pregnancies more quickly before the effects of aging take this option away completely. **Although generally well known by physicians, many couples are unaware of the profound negative effects of female age on natural and assisted reproduction.** We know that, on average, female fertility gradually declines with advancing age and becomes more pronounced after the age of 37, such that pregnancies are seldom achieved in women over the age of 42 without the use of a younger egg donor using in vitro fertilization (IVF).

An Introduction to Male Reproductive Medicine, ed. Craig Niederberger. Published by Cambridge University Press. © Cambridge University Press 2011.

If abnormalities in female reproductive function are suspected, it is entirely appropriate to refer the woman to an infertility specialist for further evaluation in conjunction with your own evaluation of the male patient. **Even in the absence of perceived abnormalities, strong consideration should be given to referring the woman over age 35 for concurrent evaluation.** The findings of that evaluation may impact the counseling you give to the couple. For example, it might be entirely appropriate to wait for 6–9 months to see an improvement in sperm counts following a varicocele repair if the female partner is 30 years of age. On the other hand, if the woman is 37 and has evidence of diminished ovarian reserve (DOR), this type of wait may have very detrimental effects on the chances for pregnancy following surgery. In this case, strong consideration may be given to proceeding directly with IVF and intracytoplasmic injection.

In the following sections, evaluation of the female partner will be discussed, emphasizing clinical factors that might give you clues on the need for a referral.

What is the definition of infertility?

Infertility is commonly defined as the lack of pregnancy following 12 months of unprotected intercourse. Couples with no infertility problems have a monthly pregnancy rate of 20–25% following properly timed intercourse. Therefore, it is not uncommon for couples to take several months to conceive a pregnancy. However, approximately 90% of couples will conceive a pregnancy by 1 year and, if this has not happened, an evaluation for possible reasons is warranted.

Conditions that warrant evaluation even before 1 year of trying to conceive:
1. Woman's age greater than 35.
2. Very irregular menstrual cycles.
3. Past history of pelvic inflammatory disease, extensive pelvic surgery, or known severe endometriosis.

Causes of infertility

To conceive a pregnancy naturally, there are several requirements. First, motile sperm must be deposited near the cervix through intercourse. Next, the sperm must be able to ascend through the cervix, uterus, and fallopian tubes, arriving at the same time a woman has released an egg (ovulated). Fertilization usually occurs near the end of the fallopian tube and the fertilized egg (embryo) is then transported over several days into the uterine cavity. Finally, the embryo must be able to implant into endometrium, which lines the uterus.

Infertility can result from a disruption in any of these normal events. Therefore, in addition to low sperm counts or motility, infertility can be due to sexual dysfunction, a lack of ovulation (anovulation), blocked fallopian tubes, or inability of an embryo to implant and establish a pregnancy in the uterus. Often there is just one problem, but sometimes infertility results from combinations of several problems.

Sexual dysfunction

When evaluating the infertile couple, a careful sexual history is important, focusing on the frequency and timing of intercourse. Problems including impotence, premature ejaculation, and dyspareunia can all lead to inadequate exposure to sperm at the time of ovulation. In addition, I have encountered many women who were uncertain of the optimal fertile time during the reproductive cycle for intercourse. We generally advise women to time intercourse around the time of ovulation (typically days 13–15 in a woman having a 28-day cycle). Alternatively, ovulation predictor kits can be used to more accurately determine the day of ovulation for timing purposes. Painful intercourse can lead to avoidance or even inability to have sex. In addition, dyspareunia may lead to a clue to other pelvic conditions contributing to infertility, including pelvic infections or endometriosis. Sometimes intercourse is infrequent due to either marital discord or lives simply being too busy, in either case, referral for counseling may be appropriate.

Ovarian dysfunction

What is a normal ovulatory cycle?

Each month, a pool of eggs is selected to enter the final growth phase of development with each egg in an ovarian follicle. The number in this pool varies but may average about 10–12 follicles out of which one is selected to become dominant and ovulate at mid-cycle whereas the others degenerate. **Commonly, ovulation occurs about day 14 of the menstrual cycle (day 1 is the first day of menstrual bleeding) but the length of the follicular growth phase can be somewhat variable, normally between 10 and 20 days.** Once the follicle is mature and ready for ovulation, luteinizing hormone (LH) is released from the pituitary gland in a mid-cycle surge that triggers ovulation of the maturing egg. LH can be detected in the urine and is the basis behind ovulation predictor kits. Following ovulation, the ovary begins to produce progesterone, which prepares the endometrial lining of the uterus for embryo implantation if the egg is successfully fertilized. Progesterone is only produced following ovulation and therefore blood levels can be used to confirm that ovulation occurred. If a pregnancy is not established in a given month, progesterone levels drop and a new menstrual cycle begins. Typically, the progesterone that is made following ovulation will cause symptoms in the woman, including breast tenderness and bloating, known as moliminal symptoms. Therefore, an ovulatory woman will typically not only have regular menstrual periods, but will also experience symptoms of breast tenderness, bloating, and sometimes mood changes accompanying the production of progesterone.

Anovulation

How do we test for ovulation?

1. *History.* Women who have regular menstrual cycles and seldom miss a period are likely to be ovulatory, particularly if they have symptoms of bloating and breast tenderness before menstrual bleeding. In this case, it is usually safe to

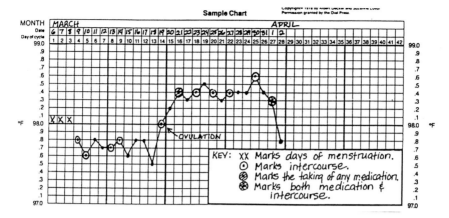

Figure 8.1 Example of a basal body temperature graph showing the rise in temperature following ovulation on day 14.

assume that the woman is ovulating and that anovulation is unlikely to be the cause of the couple's infertility. Most infertility experts will go beyond this simple history to confirm ovulation by other means.

2. *Basal body temperature graph.* For this test, a woman is asked to take her temperature first thing upon arising throughout the month. A woman's basal temperature is typically 0.5–1°F higher following ovulation (see Figure 8.1). The most fertile time of the month is just before the rise in temperature, which unfortunately can only be determined retrospectively. Many infertility experts have abandoned use of this graph as they can be difficult to interpret and emotionally difficult to keep, as they are a daily reminder to the patient of her difficulties.

3. *Urine LH-detection kits.* These kits are commercially available and require testing daily urine samples for the presence of LH. If a surge in LH is detected, ovulation is about to occur and timing for intercourse or inseminations is optimal for that day and the next day. **These tests have been shown to be quite accurate in detecting ovulation although about 7% of the time an LH surge is detected yet no ovulation occurs** [1].

4. *Serum progesterone levels.* Because progesterone is only made in high quantities following ovulation, high serum progesterone levels indicate ovulation has occurred. This test is typically obtained about 7 days after ovulation (day 21 in a typical 28-day cycle) with levels >3 ng/ml indicating ovulation. **Many infertility experts like to see progesterone levels >10 ng/ml, particularly after ovulation-inducing medication use, to indicate optimal progesterone production and fertility.**

The collapse of an ovarian follicle can be documented by serial ultrasound examinations, and histologic findings of secretory endometrium following an endometrial biopsy can also indicate that ovulation has occurred. However, these tests are not commonly utilized because of expense and discomfort.

What are common causes of anovulation?

Polycystic ovarian syndrome

The most common cause of anovulation among infertile women is polycystic ovarian syndrome (PCOS). This is a syndrome characterized by irregular menstrual cycles, some evidence of increased androgen production, and multiple small ovarian follicles detected by ultrasound. The most common complaint with PCOS is irregular menstrual periods due to anovulation. Increased hair growth ("hirsutism") with or without acne are common with PCOS, due to the effects of androgens. Most, but not all, women with PCOS are overweight, but there is a "thin variant" of PCOS as well. Patients with PCOS often have insulin resistance, which is more pronounced in obese women. Therefore, long-term health consequences of PCOS include an increased risk of diabetes, hypertension, and perhaps cardiovascular disease [2,3]. PCOS also has been linked to an increased risk of depression and endometrial cancer.

If a woman is overweight, the first step in managing PCOS is weight loss through diet and exercise. No one particular diet has been shown to be beneficial over another, rather, the important point is to restrict calories in an effort to lose weight. In general, 30 minutes or more of exercise daily in addition to regular activities is recommended. **Several studies have demonstrated that even a 10% reduction in body weight is very beneficial in establishing more regular ovulatory cycles and improving fertility** [4]. Therefore, the goal of weight loss does not need to be a return to ideal weight. Unfortunately, many women with PCOS report great difficulty in losing weight despite restricting calories and exercising faithfully.

If weight loss is difficult or fails to establish ovulatory cycles, several ovulation-inducing medications can be used to treat infertility (see section below on ovulation induction).

Elevated prolactin level

Elevations in the pituitary hormone prolactin can lead to anovulation by interrupting the pulsatile release of gonadotropin-releasing hormone. Prolactin is an important hormone for lactation and therefore some, but not all, women will note breast milk secretion when prolactin is elevated. Causes of elevated prolactin include prolactinomas, hypothyroidism, and use of some antidepressant and antihypertensive medications, among others. Because hypothyroidism can cause irregular cycles and elevated prolactin levels, both thyroid-stimulating hormone and prolactin are commonly measured in women with anovulation.

Women found to have an elevated prolactin level will need further testing to establish the cause of the elevation. Prolactin levels can then be lowered either by giving thyroid hormone replacement therapy in the case of hypothyroidism, or through the use of dopamine agonist drugs such as bromocriptine, which lower prolactin levels. Once the prolactin level is normalized, regular ovulatory cycles frequently begin and fertility is often restored.

Ovarian failure and premature menopause

Some women do not ovulate because they are menopausal (complete absence of menses) or in the menopausal transition (perimenopause). The perimenopause is characterized by menstrual irregularity in a woman who previously had regular periods and precedes true menopause by several years [5]. In the menopausal transition, menses often actually occur more frequently before they begin to space out and become more and more infrequent. Estrogen production is low leading to some of the common symptoms of menopause, including absence of periods, hot flashes, and vaginal dryness. **The average age of menopause is 51; however, some women undergo premature menopause, which is defined as menopause before the age of 40.**

Premature menopause can be caused by chromosomal problems, genetic disorders, previous ovarian surgery, previous chemotherapy or radiation therapy for cancer, and autoimmune conditions. Despite a complete evaluation, many times the cause of early ovarian failure is unknown. The diagnosis is made by clinical findings combined with an elevated FSH level. The only treatment that is highly effective at this time is the use of donor eggs and IVF.

Stress-induced amenorrhea

Some women will not ovulate or menstruate due to physical or psychological stress. This type of anovulation is also called "hypothalamic amenorrhea" because stress inhibits the secretion of gonadotropin-releasing hormone in the hypothalamus, which, in turn, causes a "shut-down" of the reproductive cycle and anovulation. The most common source of stress is excessive exercise combined with weight loss or low body weight. Women with anorexia nervosa fall into this category of anovulation. **This cause of anovulation is often a diagnosis of exclusion after other causes are ruled out; however, low FSH levels in conjunction with low body weight are highly suggestive.**

Women with stress-induced amenorrhea are encouraged to reduce exercise and gain weight. If successful, regular ovulatory cycles usually resume. Sometimes weight gain is difficult and then ovulation-inducing medications can be prescribed. Available oral medications are less successful in women with this type of anovulation and often injectable gonadotropin therapy, including both LH and FSH, are required to stimulate ovulation.

Obesity-related anovulation

Sometimes overweight patients will not meet the criteria for PCOS yet will have anovulation, perhaps due to tonically high estrogen levels from the aromatization of androgens by fat. This leads to inappropriate suppression of ovulation at the hypothalamic–pituitary axis. These women will be aided by weight loss or use of ovulation-induction medications.

Ovarian insufficiency or "diminished ovarian reserve"

Another cause of infertility is ovarian insufficiency, also known as diminished ovarian reserve (DOR). **DOR is known to be more common in older reproductive age women and it can be difficult to diagnose by history alone.** Women with DOR often still have regular menses. However, when stimulated with gonadotropins, these women produce fewer eggs and this can result in lower pregnancy rates with infertility treatments.

Unlike the testicle where stem cells replenish spermatozoa continuously, there are no stem cells in the ovary to replenish egg supplies. Thus, women are born with a set number of eggs that does not increase over time, and, in fact, declines at variable rates [5]. **With aging, there is a decline not only in egg number but also egg quality, which is thought to be largely due to chromosomal abnormalities.** The chromosomal problems, in turn, cause reduced fertility, increased risk of miscarriage, and increased risk of having a child with chromosomal problems, such as trisomy 21.

How do we diagnose diminished ovarian reserve?

1. *Day 3 FSH.* The most common test for decreased ovarian reserve is a day 3 FSH and estradiol level [6]. FSH elevated above 12 mIU/ml indicates DOR. Estradiol levels are commonly measured at the same time and values should be less than 80 pg/ml on cycle day 3. If estradiol levels are above this level, they can lead to a falsely diminished FSH level and reduce the accuracy of FSH determination.
2. *Ultrasound measures.* DOR can also be suggested by transvaginal ultrasound observation of the ovaries. Women with DOR have small ovaries with decreased ovarian volume (<3 cm^3) and decreased numbers of ovarian follicles measuring between 2 and 9 mm in diameter. This number is called the antral follicle count and totals less than 10 (combination of both ovaries) suggest DOR.
3. *Anti-Müllerian hormone levels.* **Anti-Müllerian hormone is only made by early ovarian follicles and blood levels of this hormone have been shown to correlate with the number of eggs present within the ovaries.** The exact level of hormone used to diagnose DOR may vary depending on the laboratory used. However, one study has shown that a level under 1.25 ng/ml is highly sensitive for detecting women with DOR [7].

Limitations of testing

We truly do not have ideal tests for DOR at this time. All the currently available tests are better at estimating egg number and do not tell us about egg quality, which ultimately may be more important for fertility. Therefore, the tests are better at predicting who has a higher risk of having an IVF cycle cancelled for inadequate egg numbers than in predicting who will or will not get pregnant from a cycle. In addition, all tests have less than ideal sensitivity and specificity leading to false reassurance in some cases and false alarm in others. The problem of false diagnosis of DOR is worse among younger patients. Therefore, at this time, these tests should only be used as indicators of a possible problem and should seldom be used to exclude patients from trying an infertility treatment.

Treatment

Most infertility experts will advise women who are suspected of having DOR to move forward with more "aggressive" infertility treatments. These include use of ovulation induction with gonadotropin injections or IVF (see below). Ultimately, if DOR is confirmed by a lack of ovarian responsiveness to medications, use of donor eggs is often required. Even so, some women diagnosed with DOR will still conceive naturally.

Tubal disease/pelvic adhesive disease

Another cause of infertility is damaged fallopian tubes or pelvic adhesions surrounding the fallopian tube and ovary.

Normal physiology
After ovulation, the fallopian tube moves across the surface of the ovary and captures the released egg. If the fallopian tube is open, sperm can ascend the female reproductive tract and fertilize the egg at the end of the tube. Cilia within the tube propel the early embryo towards the uterine cavity over approximately 5 days and the embryo is then capable of attaching to and implanting into the endometrium. The fallopian tube must be open and free of adhesive disease in order to serve these functions. Pelvic adhesions may interfere with egg capture as well as sperm and embryo transport predisposing to infertility or an ectopic pregnancy.

What can lead to damaged fallopian tubes or pelvic adhesions?

Sexually transmitted infections. The most common cause of damaged fallopian tubes is previous sexually transmitted infection, including gonorrhea and chlamydia. These organisms are known to ascend the female reproductive tract and infect the fallopian tubes leading to pelvic pain and fever in the short term, early and tubal damage and adhesions in the long term. **Sometimes a history of an infection is known, but the infections can be asymptomatic. Chlamydia, in particular, can often cause few symptoms yet tubal damage can be severe.**

Other infections. It is also possible for other bacteria to ascend the reproductive tract and cause pelvic adhesions. In addition, appendicitis, particularly if the appendix ruptures, can damage fallopian tubes.

Previous pelvic surgery. Pelvic surgeries on the fallopian tubes (ectopic pregnancy, tubal ligation), ovaries (removal of ovarian cysts, including endometriomas), or uterus (myomectomy) can lead to scarring in the pelvis. Significant bowel surgery for ulcerative colitis, Crohn's disease, or infections such as appendicitis or diverticulitis can cause scarring and tubal damage.

Endometriosis can also cause tubal obstruction and pelvic adhesions. Endometriosis is further discussed in the following sections.

How are fallopian tubes tested?

1. *Hysterosalpingogram* (HSG) is the most common radiologic test used to determine tubal anatomy by injecting contrast through the cervix into the uterus and fallopian tubes and observing under fluoroscopy. Following injection, contrast can be observed spilling from the end of the fallopian tube into the peritoneal cavity, indicating patency (Figure 8.2). The tubes may also be blocked either distally or proximally. A tube that is greatly dilated and filled with fluid is called a hydrosalpinx. Some clinics determine tubal patency by injecting saline through the cervix and observing flow of saline through the tubes by ultrasound.

2. *Laparoscopy* is occasionally warranted to evaluate tubal patency by directly observing dye exiting the fallopian tube after being injected through the cervix. This surgical procedure is being used with less and less frequency for evaluating infertility due to its high cost and invasive nature.

What is the best treatment for tubal damage?

If fallopian tubes are badly damaged, the best modern treatment is IVF, which has the advantage of "bypassing" them entirely. **If hydrosalpinges are present, studies have shown that removing the tubes entirely leads to improved pregnancy rates with IVF** [8]. With less severe adhesive disease, surgical resection by laparoscopy is a reasonable option that may improve fertility, although adhesion re-formation is a concern.

If a couple desires a pregnancy following a tubal ligation, tubal ligation reversal can be considered. Some types of tubal ligations cannot be successfully reversed and the presence of other infertility factors must be assessed. **However, if a couple is a good candidate for surgery, tubal ligation reversal is associated with about a 90% tubal patency rate and a 50–60% chance of conceiving a baby in 1 year.** These benefits must be weighed against the risks of having a surgical procedure and a 5–10% chance of having an ectopic (tubal) pregnancy following the reversal. An attractive alternative treatment is IVF for these couples.

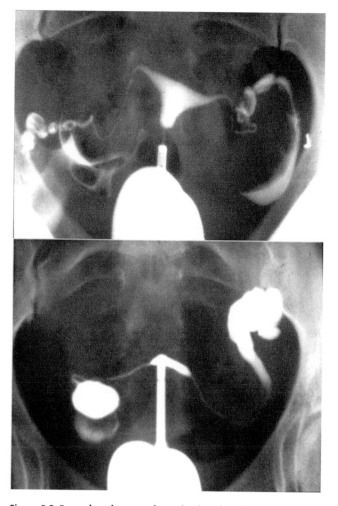

Figure 8.2 Examples of a normal HSG (top) with spill of contrast from the tubes and an abnormal HSG (bottom) with dilated tubes and no free spill of contrast.

Endometriosis

Endometriosis is a pathologic condition in which endometrial glands are growing in the peritoneal cavity. During a normal menstrual period, the endometrium is sloughed and exits the cervix and vagina with menses. However, some of the sloughed endometrium also refluxes through the fallopian tubes and can attach and grow in the pelvic peritoneal surface – causing endometriosis. Common sites for endometriosis are in the cul-de-sac as well as around the fallopian tubes and ovaries. Endometriosis causes infertility and pelvic pain, which commonly worsens around the time of the menstrual period.

Endometriosis can vary both in amount of disease and severity of symptoms. Mild endometriosis is characterized by small implants of tissue causing essentially no distortion of pelvic anatomy. The pathophysiology of infertility is not clear with minimal endometriosis. Severe endometriosis can essentially invade any organ in the pelvis leading to blood-filled ovarian cysts (endometriomas) and great amounts of scarring that disrupt the fallopian tubes. In this case, infertility may be caused by distortion of the normal anatomy.

For many cases of endometriosis, presence of the disease can be suggested by pain symptoms and findings on pelvic or ultrasound examination. However, the only way to diagnose endometriosis with certainty is by laparoscopy. When extensive endometriosis is suggested by pain symptoms or pelvic exam, laparoscopy is warranted both to diagnose and treat the disease, as this will likely improve both pain and infertility. **In the absence of pain symptoms or abnormal findings on exam, laparoscopy is not necessary as treatment of minimal disease has not been shown to improve fertility either minimally or not at all and, ultimately, IVF is a more cost-effective approach** [9].

Uterine factor infertility

Occasionally, abnormalities of the uterus are thought to contribute to infertility. These lesions are most often diagnosed by ultrasound examination of the pelvis.

Fibroids (myomas leiomyomas), are very common smooth muscle tumors of the uterus. Because fibroids are so common, it is difficult to know if the fibroids are actually causing the infertility or if they are merely present but having no impact on fertility. **Most infertility experts will consider fibroids to be the cause of infertility only if all other factors have been ruled out.** Fibroids located next to the endometrial lining of the uterus have the biggest impact on fertility and are often removed surgically [10].

Endometrial polyps are small growths of the endometrium, which are usually benign in premenopausal women. Larger polyps tend to persist and there is some evidence that removing these by surgery improves fertility.

Inadequate endometrial development or "luteal phase defect"

Progesterone is critical for implantation and pregnancy. Some have theorized that inadequate progesterone production is a cause of infertility. For many years, infertility experts recommended that an endometrial biopsy be done to look for poor development of the endometrium. More recently, studies suggest that an endometrial biopsy should seldom be performed during the infertility evaluation. **A recent large study found that poorly developed endometrial or "luteal phase defect" was present just as often in fertile women as it is in infertile women raising questions as to whether this truly is a cause of infertility** [11].

In addition, interpretation of the endometrial biopsy is quite difficult and varies significantly from one pathologist to another. It may still be that inadequate endometrial development is a factor causing infertility, but we may not have good means of testing for this.

Cervical factor infertility

Throughout most of the cycle, cervical mucus is thick and slows sperm from ascending the female reproductive tract. Around mid-cycle, when ovulation occurs, cervical mucus increases in amount and thins out allowing sperm to more readily ascend the female reproductive tract. Abnormal cervical mucus may contribute to infertility if it is too thick, or decreased in amount, particularly after surgery to the cervix. Cervical mucus might become abnormally thick as a side-effect of the ovulation-inducing medication, clomiphene citrate (see below). Although clomiphene citrate has beneficial effects on ovulation, it can have negative effects on cervical mucus production and thickness. Infections in the vagina and cervix could theoretically have effects on sperm function and ascent, although this is less proven.

Cervical mucus is evaluated by the post-coital test, which is performed by obtaining a cervical mucus sample at mid-cycle several hours following inter-course. The presence of motile sperm can be detected by microscopic examin-ation of the cervical mucus. This test has fallen out of favor because of lack of standardization of the test and because the common treatment for an abnormal test, intrauterine insemination (IUI), is often used even when the test is normal. In other words, the results do not often change the management.

Summary of the infertility evaluation

Usually, infertility specialists will investigate all common causes of infertility with the following tests:
1. Day 21 progesterone level – detects ovulation.
2. Seminal fluid analysis.
3. Hysterosalpingogram.
4. Pelvic ultrasound and ovarian reserve testing in some women.

Unexplained infertility

Despite a thorough work-up, at least 25–30% of couples will have no obvious explanation for their infertility, resulting in a diagnosis of unexplained infertility. Although this diagnosis can be quite frustrating to couples, it is reassuring to note that pregnancy rates with treatments in couples with this disorder are as good or better following treatment as compared with those where a diagnosis is established.

Infertility treatments

The recommended treatments will, of course, vary depending on the cause. In certain instances (tubal damage, severe endometriosis, fibroids, and polyps), surgery will be recommended. With many other causes of infertility, the basic concept is to increase the number of eggs and sperm at the site of fertilization to improve the chances of conceiving a pregnancy. These treatments fall under the categories of ovulation induction and insemination used either alone or in combination. IVF is being used with increasing frequency for all types of infertility as success rates continue to improve with this treatment.

Ovulation-induction medications

Oral medications
Clomiphene citrate is commonly used to enhance ovulation in women who are either anovulatory or women who are already ovulating but not getting pregnant. The medication is very effective in women who are not ovulating but there are only small beneficial effects in women who are already ovulating.

With clomiphene citrate, a starting dose is chosen (typically 50 or 100 mg) and given for 5 days starting on cycle days 3–5 (day 1 is the first day of menstrual bleeding). To detect ovulation, women can use a urine LH detection kit but this should not start before day 11 of the cycle as the drug can cause a false-positive reading. Often, progesterone levels on day 21 are also measured. Sometimes the dose needs to be adjusted up if ovulation does not occur with initial doses. Common side-effects include: hot flashes, mood swings, mild pelvic discomfort, and multiple birth (twins 8–10% chance, <1% chance of triplets or more).

Other oral medications for ovulation induction include tamoxifen, a drug similar to clomiphene citrate in its actions. The aromatase inhibitor letrozole (Femara) has also been used for ovulation induction, although this drug is not Food and Drug Administration approved for this purpose. Finally, metformin (Glucophage) can be used in women with PCOS. Metformin improves insulin sensitivity and, when used alone, has only a modest effect in increasing ovulation. **Sometimes metformin is combined with clomiphene citrate for ovulation induction, although a recent large study found that this drug combination was no more effective than clomiphene citrate alone in a large population of women with PCOS** [12]. Nevertheless, there may be some women who are not ovulating on clomiphene citrate alone who will ovulate in response to the combination of these drugs.

Injectable drugs for ovulation induction

Gonadotropin injections
Another option for inducing ovulation in women is the use of gonadotropin (LH and FSH) injections. These medications are given by daily injections and they act by directly stimulating ovarian follicular development and ovulation.

They are expensive and require careful monitoring by ultrasound due to the significantly increased risk of ovarian hyperstimulation and multiple gestations as compared with oral medications. Sometimes oral medications are given first, followed by injectable gonadotropins. This combination can reduce the number of injections needed and reduces the total amount of gonadotropin drugs used and, therefore, cost of treatment. Pregnancy rates are similar to gonadotropins alone [13].

Intrauterine insemination (IUI)

IUI is a commonly used treatment for infertility. The basic concept is that with natural intercourse many sperm never ascend the female reproductive tract because they are lost out of the vagina or never make it past the cervical mucus. With IUI, a semen sample is brought to the laboratory when the female partner is ovulating. This sample is then processed so the motile sperm are isolated and concentrated from the ejaculate. The concentrated sperm are then placed past the cervix into the uterus through a small catheter.

IUI is indicated for cases of unexplained infertility, cervical factor infertility, and mild male factor infertility. **IUI is much less effective when there are severe male factor problems defined by low numbers of motile sperm in the ejaculate (<10 million motile sperm) or in the prepared sample to be placed into the uterus (<1 million motile sperm).** IUI is also commonly utilized in conjunction with ovulation-induction medications as pregnancy rates are improved as compared with using these treatments separately [14].

What pregnancy rates can be expected from various treatments?

Pregnancy rates with different treatments will vary depending on the cause of infertility and the woman's age. Rates that might be expected in a 35-year-old woman with unexplained infertility are shown in Table 8.1.

In vitro fertilization

IVF has the highest pregnancy rates of any infertility treatment [15]. However, it is also the most involved and expensive of the treatments so usually other treatments are attempted first for most causes of infertility.

Steps in the in vitro fertilization process

1. Ovarian stimulation is done with combinations of injectable drugs for several weeks. The goal is to get many follicles developing so that eggs can be retrieved. Figure 8.3A shows an ultrasound view of an unstimulated ovary. Figure 8.3B is the same ovary after several days of stimulation. The black ovals in the figure are fluid-filled ovarian follicles that contain eggs.

Table 8.1 Outcomes to expect from common infertility treatments

	Delivery rate/cycle	Multiple birth rate/pregnancy
Timed intercourse	2–3%	1%
IUI alone	5%	1%
Clomid alone	5%	10%
Clomid and IUI	8%	10%
hMG alone	12%–15%	15%
hMG and IUI	15%–18%	15%
In vitro fertilization[a]	30–32%	31%

[a]Based on 2008 national data from SART.
hMG, human menopausal gonadotropin; IUI, intrauterine insemination.

2. Once the eggs are thought to be mature based on ultrasound measurements of the follicles, egg retrieval is performed under ultrasound guidance (Figure 8.3C). This step is performed with sedatives and pain medications.
3. The retrieved eggs (Figure 8.3D) are next fertilized in the laboratory, either by mixing eggs with sperm in a culture dish (E) or by injecting a single sperm into the egg (F) by a process called intracytoplasmic injection.
4. The resulting embryos are then cultured for several days (Figure 8.3G is a 3-day-old 8-cell embryo and H is a 5-day-old blastocyst embryo) before the best embryos are selected to be transferred back to the uterus (I).
5. Extra embryos of good quality are frozen for later use if needed.

Outcomes

Outcomes are very dependent on the age of the woman being stimulated. In addition, different centers have different pregnancy rates dependent, in part, on the populations of patients they are treating. Because some centers may treat mainly older patients or patients who have had IVF failures elsewhere ("tougher patients"), it is difficult to directly compare centers. However, age-specific outcomes from various centers are available on the internet.

Other treatments available with in vitro fertilization include

- *Preimplantation genetic diagnosis* – used to avoid genetic diseases in offspring.
- *Preimplantation genetic screening* – used to screen for chromosomal abnormalities in embryos in the hope of decreasing the pregnancy loss rate and perhaps increasing the pregnancy rate. In Figure 8.4, a single cell is removed from an eight-cell embryo (A). The cell is then analyzed for the numbers of chromosomes present using color-coded probes (B). In this case, the presence of three bright red probes indicates that there is an extra, abnormal chromosome instead of the expected number of two chromosomes.

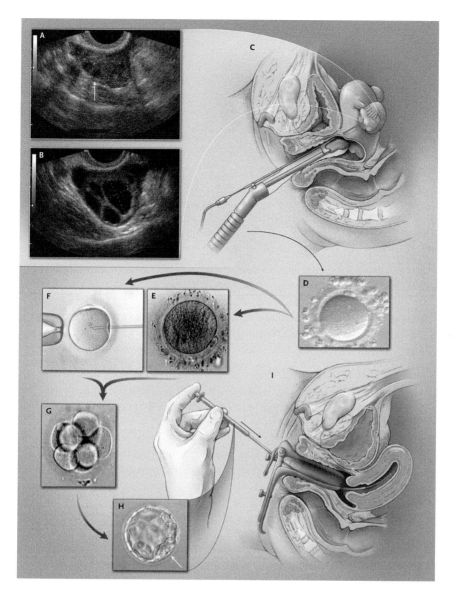

Figure 8.3 Steps in the IVF process: 1. Ovarian stimulation is done with combinations of injectable drugs for several weeks. The goal is to get many follicles developing so that eggs can be retrieved. In the figure above, A shows an ultrasound view of an unstimulated ovary. B is the same ovary after several days of stimulation. The black ovals are fluid-filled ovarian follicles that contain eggs. 2. Once the eggs are thought to be mature based on ultrasound measurements of the follicles, egg retrieval is performed under ultrasound guidance (C). This step is performed with sedatives and pain medications. 3. The retrieved eggs (D) are next fertilized in the laboratory, either by mixing eggs with sperm in a culture dish (E) or by injecting a single sperm into the egg (F) by a process called intracytoplasmic injection. 4. The resulting embryos are then cultured for several days (G is a 3-day-old eight-cell embryo, H is a 5-day-old blastocyst embryo) before the best embryos are selected to be transferred back to the uterus(I) (see color plate section).

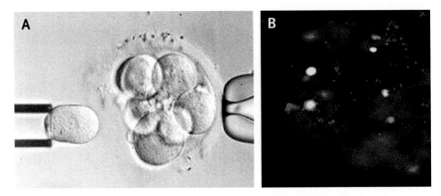

Figure 8.4 Preimplantation genetic screening (PGS) – used to screen for chromosomal abnormalities in embryos to decrease the pregnancy loss rate and possibly increase the pregnancy rate. In the figure above, a single cell is removed from an eight-cell embryo (A). The cell is then analyzed for the numbers of chromosomes present using color-coded probes (B). In this case, the presence of three bright red probes indicates that there is an extra, abnormal chromosome instead of the expected number of two chromosomes. (See color plate section).

- *Donor eggs or embryos* – used mainly in couples where the woman does not produce sufficient numbers of good-quality eggs. Depending on donor age, high pregnancy rates are seen with this treatment.
- *Cryopreserved embryo transfer* – often, extra embryos from the "fresh" IVF cycle are frozen for later use. These embryos can be thawed and transferred back to the uterus. Although pregnancy rates are generally somewhat lower than in the fresh cycle, these cycles have the advantage of being less expensive.
- *Surrogacy*– hiring another woman who will have embryos transferred and carry the pregnancy.
- *Egg freezing* – a new technique that is currently experimental. The goal of this treatment is to hopefully preserve a woman's fertility into the future.

Lifestyle recommendations for improved fertility [16]

1. Stop smoking: cigarette smoking reduces the monthly chance for natural conception in all large studies.
2. Women should try to adjust diet and exercise to maintain a body mass index of between 20 kg/m^2 and 27 kg/m^2.
3. Both partners should limit alcohol intake to no more than four drinks/week. Once pregnant, all alcohol consumption by the woman should stop.
4. Female partners should limit caffeine intake to no more than 250 mg/day (approximately two cups of coffee a day). Caffeine intake higher than this has been associated with increased time to conceive.

5. Exercise for more than 60 min/day is associated with an increased prevalence of anovulation. Therefore, it is probably wise to use this as a limit while trying to conceive.

REFERENCES

[1] McGovern PG, Myers ER, Silva S, *et al.* NICHD National Cooperative Reproductive Medicine Network. Absence of secretory endometrium after false-positive home urine luteinizing hormone testing. *Fertil Steril* 2004; **82**: 1273–7.

[2] Legro RS. A 27-year-old woman with a diagnosis of polycystic ovary syndrome. *JAMA* 2007; **297**: 509–19.

[3] Shroff R, Syrop CH, Davis W, *et al.* Risk of metabolic complications in the new PCOS phenotypes based on the Rotterdam criteria. *Fertil Steril* 2007; **88**: 1389–95.

[4] Norman RJ, Dewailly D, Legro RS, Hickey TE. Polycystic ovary syndrome. *Lancet* 2007; **370**: 685–97.

[5] Santoro N. The menopausal transition. *Am J Med* 2005; **118**: 8–13.

[6] Bancsi LF, Broekmans FJ, Mol BW, Habbema JD, te Velde ER. Performance of basal follicle-stimulating hormone in the prediction of poor ovarian response and failure to become pregnant after in vitro fertilization: a meta-analysis. *Fertil Steril* 2003; **79**: 1091–100.

[7] La Marca A, Sighinolfi G, Radu D, *et al.* Anti-Mullerian hormone (AMH) as a predictive marker in assisted reproductive technology (ART). *Hum Reprod Update* 2010; **16**(2): 113–30.

[8] Strandell A, Lindhard A, Waldenström U, Thorburn J. Hydrosalpinx and IVF outcome: cumulative results after salpingectomy in a randomized controlled trial. *Hum Reprod* 2001; **16**: 2403–10.

[9] Van Voorhis BJ, Stovall DW, Allen BD, Syrop CH. Cost-effective treatment of the infertile couple. *Fertil Steril* 1998; **70**: 995–1005.

[10] Pritts EA, Parker WH, Olive DL. Fibroids and infertility: an updated systematic review of the evidence. *Fertil Steril* 2009; **91**: 1215–23.

[11] Coutifaris C, Myers ER, Guzick DS, *et al.* NICHD National Cooperative Reproductive Medicine Network. Histological dating of timed endometrial biopsy tissue is not related to fertility status. *Fertil Steril* 2004; **82**: 1264–72.

[12] Legro RS, Barnhart HX, Schlaff WD, *et al.* Cooperative Multicenter Reproductive Medicine Network. Clomiphene, metformin, or both for infertility in the polycystic ovary syndrome. *N Engl J Med* 2007; **356**: 551–66.

[13] Ryan GL, Moss V, Davis WA, *et al.* Oral ovulation induction agents combined with low-dose gonadotropin injections and intrauterine insemination: cost- and clinical effectiveness. *J Reprod Med* 2005; **50**: 943–50.

[14] Van Voorhis BJ, Barnett M, Sparks AE, *et al.* Effect of the total motile sperm count on the efficacy and cost-effectiveness of intrauterine insemination and in vitro fertilization. *Fertil Steril* 2001; **75**: 661–8.

[15] Van Voorhis BJ. Clinical practice. In vitro fertilization. *N Engl J Med* 2007; **356**: 379–86.

[16] Barbieri RL. The initial fertility consultation: recommendations concerning cigarette smoking, body mass index, and alcohol and caffeine consumption. *Am J Obstet Gynecol* 2001; **185**: 1168–73.

Index

Printed in the United States
by Baker & Taylor Publisher Services